# THE STRONGEST MAN THAT EVER LIVED

(ORIGINAL VERSION, RESTORED)

By

## GEORGE F. JOWETT

FOUNDER AND PRESIDENT OF THE AMERICAN CONTINENTAL
WEIGHT LIFTERS' ASSOCIATION ONE OF THE WORLD'S
STRONGEST ATHLETES AND AUTHOR OF "THE KEY TO MIGHT
AND MUSCLE."

Originally Published in 1927

PUBLISHED BY O'Faolain Patriot LLC, Copyright 2011
info@PhysicalCultureBooks.com
Published in the United States of America

ISBN-13: 978-1466442771

ISBN-10: 1466442778

# TABLEOFCONTENTS

# PREFACE

When I took up my pen to write "The Key to Might and Muscle" I did so because I desired to tell you of many things that others had missed, or overlooked in their various, explorations of "the magnificent man." I wanted to open before you the lessons that life had taught me by placing "the key" in your hands. I feel that I have done it, yet while languishing from my labors, to my mind came another thought, as I visioned a space that checked my musings. I perceived that my duty to my circle of body lovers was not fulfilled. There was another task ahead and I must do something different to completely fill the aurora of the body lovers' landscape—I took up my pen and wrote this book of a song of secret aspirations, which through all the years of my life of toil has been the font that fibred my existence. For many, many years I have worshipped in silence at the altar of the god-like man, and pressed the nectar of inspiration that poured from them to my lips. I felt its warm glow of cleanliness course through the veins like wine through the blood. It felt like band music going by. A spontaneous sort of rapture that makes the eye quick, and the speech incoherent, but the muscles throb vibrantly.

I am at the age in life when we are told that labor and joy mixed with the tears of happiness mellows our judgment, brings us levity and makes our ideals earthy. Happily, the former is true, but positively not the latter if you still have courage. For myself, I remain just the same, inasmuch as that I still see the gods that I enshrined upon their pedestals of a purity far richer than the gold dross of this world. Theirs is the vast splendor of manly beauty and physical purity, encased with indomitable strength. Each one a living, breathing ideal, though made of clay, fashioned of God.

Who dare say that my creed is wrong, while all around us we see the world enslaved in dissipation to its creed of gold. Completely forgotten to them is the house that God built. Then what right has any to deny us the privilege to pay tribute to our idealism, which stands like Moses on the Mount—undefiled.

So, dear strength lover, because my creed is yours, I have drawn together the golden threads of a great man's life and spun the web of his story within these pages. The manner in which this book is written is entirely a new departure in strong-man journalism. I have bared my soul and purposely scorned the reins of conventional writing by giving full sway to my exultations, and perhaps to a few lamentations, but not many, as there is so little reason for them, especially when we consider that all things happen for the best. If I have in places appeared too abandon and let the fire of my song run riot, forgive me, remember I am human and that my strength is my weakness, for I love the God-made man even as you do.

As you read through these pages, I hope you will feel the throbs of excitement that I have lived. The straining at the leash of a restless spirit as mine has been, the enveloping passion to shout and hurl sky-high your hat like a baseball fan, as you visualize our hero crash through the battle line to victory. I want you to see this man as I have seen him, sweaty, palpitating, sometimes bloody, but with a triumphant eye as he looked over his battlefields.

I only hope you will like this book and inspire others to possess it, so that this volume will be the first of many to fire your soul and urge you to beautify your body even as my other book so instructs and guides.

Strongly yours,
The Author, GEORGE F. JOWETT.

# CHAPTER I

Quebec! Beautiful Quebec! What a pageant of thoughts surge through my mind as the six little letters which compose that magic word drip from my pen. One great writer named it the "enchanted province," thinking only of its natural beauty, as did Champlain nigh three hundred years ago when he wrote his royal master at Versailles of the new colony, "La belle du France." The spell of beauty sprinkled its mist over this glorified province long before the great Cartier sailed up the majestic St. Lawrence, to cast the first anchor in the St. Charles River.

The spell has remained, to grow and remain always as a thing apart, more entrancing even than Longfellow's land of Evangeline. Its barbaric splendor rears its rugged head like a mighty queen who fosters no weaklings, bequeathing her earthly womb as a cradle of strong men.

Such has her brood been, men who thrilled to pit their powers against the elements of God or man, with a resolution that despised pain. Turn the pages of history and see the array of dauntless men who thrust forward the march of progress, with a fearless tread, far beyond the Mississippi, facing hunger, thirst, torture and death with iron courage and unshakeable faith in the cross that each man bore. Each episode reviewed in its respective light of conquest, my sympathies and admiration are drawn to the little band of descendants of the followers of Cartier, who swore their fealty to that magnificent lord of chivalry and physical might, Maisenneauve; the man who slew the great Huron chieftain whose prowess was chanted in all the wigwams far towards the setting sun. In a hand-to-hand encounter on the site of Place d'Armes, Maisenneauve won the land by right of might upon which the site and surroundings of Montreal now stand.

His followers were the hardiest of all the hardy adventurers, and it is only fitting that from this group should descend the man whose great feats of physical prowess assured his immortality among men—Louis Cyr, the man who for many years has been termed the "daddy of 'em all;" a colossal pillar of strength with a heart as big as his soul, which imparted good fellowship and geniality upon all who came within the sunshine of his smile. In reproof he was very mild, as Goldsmith would say, "More destined to guide than chide." He recognized his great strength and the frailty of others in comparison, which probably was the reason why he could forbear and become more tolerable with others, as was certainly always the case with him. Is there any wonder that around such a character a deep feeling of respect should have been established? In his native province he was followed with a dog-like devotion of adoration that enshrined him on the altar of demigods. Probably it was not the Carlyle kind of hero worship, for their creed is too simple but utterly unshakeable—the creed of the French Canadian.

When I ponder over the characteristics of Louis Cyr, I realize how humble one so great can be before God and man and yet so exalted. Then I find more depth in Gray's "Elegy" and eulogy to man.

Much confusion surrounds the exact birthplace of the nineteenth century Samson. I have seen no less than five different spots claimed as the cradle of "Our Louis." He first saw the light of day on the eleventh of October, 1863, in the little village of St. Cyprien, Quebec, and was born of parents who had been tillers of the soil and hardy woodsmen for generations. Although his father was a powerful, stockily built man, it is to his mother that he owes an ancestry of prodigious super-men. Tremendously formed, the mother of this great son evoked more awe and admiration than her mighty offspring. Terrifically strong, she stood six feet one inch and weighed two hundred and sixty- seven pounds in her prime. Looming out of the wild primeval setting of Quebec, a mighty Amazon above all others, with piercing eye and commanding carriage, the son she bore was a just tribute to her forebears. She reminds me of what her ancient Gaulish ancestors must have been, when the women followed their men into battle and slew with a berserk fury that must have been appalling. Being women of steel fiber, they equaled their warrior husbands in withstanding hardships. Such was her race, and, probably, she was the last of her kind. Many a tree fell before the onslaught of her axe as the land was cleared and winter fuel brought in. In such a vigorous atmosphere was young Louis reared, and with each succeeding year his form filled out into the sturdiness of the oak. When he crept into his 'teens he was above the average man for strength and already manifested a love to display his great natural powers.

The story is told that one day as he journeyed home along the old dirt trails of those days, he came upon a straining team of horses, who were struggling to draw their load from out of a deep rut into which the wheels had sunk; but neither failing strength stimulated under the lash of the whip, nor the exhortations of the teamster could move the load. As Louis neared the scene he saw a team of horses trembling from their exertions, and a voluble French teamster standing helplessly by.

"M'sier, M'sier," young Louis reprimanded, "You should not abuse your horses that way."

"But I cannot stay here all night with my load. It has to be drawn out," the teamster replied. "What am I to do," he wailed. "They cannot move it."

"Oh! M'sier, but you take the wrong method," Louis answered. "I will show you how."

Then, before the astonished eyes of the teamster, the youthful descendant of a Gaulish chieftain got under the back of the wagon and placed his hands upon his knees, while his back strained up against the load. Inch by inch the wagon wheels rose, until they were clear of the rut; then with a side movement the load was transferred out of the rut onto the road level. Louis beamed with pleasure on the success of Montgomery Irving, a beautifully built Englishman who linked his fortune with Cyclops on their American invasion. He bore a great resemblance to Eugene Sandow, and because he added the letter e to Sandow and toured as Sandowe, he became known as "the false Sandowe."

Horace Barre, who as a boy played a part in the unmasking of Cyclops and the false Sandowe by defeating the latter as easily as Cyr defeated the former. Barre grew to be terrifically strong, and in my mind at that time stood next in rank to his great teammate, Louis Cyr, on the question of strength.

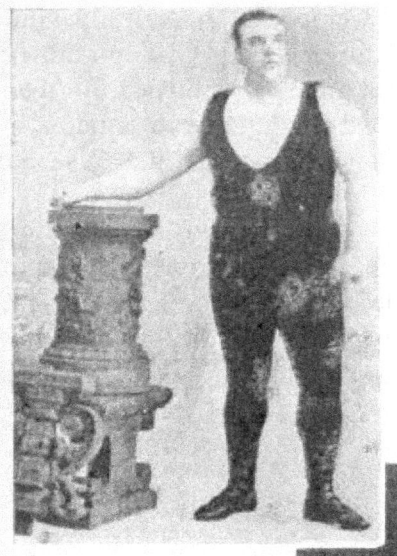

Horace Barre, who as a boy played a part in the unmasking of Cyclops and the false Sandowe by defeating the latter as easily as Cyr defeated the former. Barre grew to be terrifically strong, and in my mind at that time stood next in rank to his great teammate, Louis Cyr, on the question of strength.

Montgomery Irving, a beautifully built Englishman who linked his fortune with Cyclops on their American invasion. He bore a great resemblance to Eugene S a n d o w, a n d because he added the letter e to S a n d o w and toured as Sandowe, he became known as "the f a l s e Sandowe."

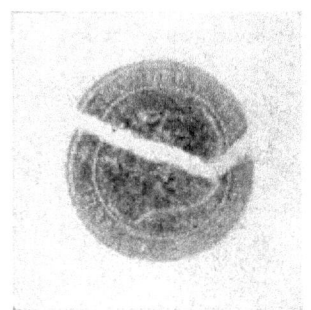

An actual reproduction of a coin broken by Cyclops.

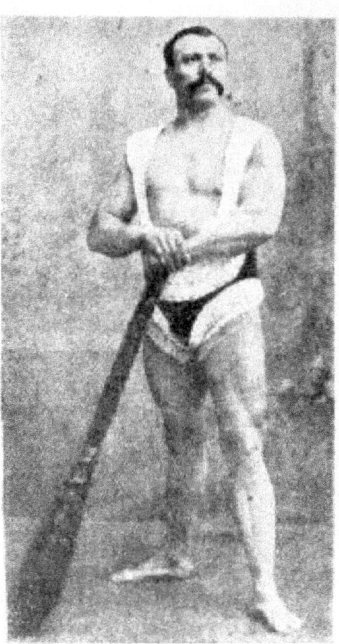

Noel, a French strong man, who lost on a coin-breaking test to Cyclops.

Cyclops had wonderful finger strength. He never had any difficulty in breaking coins between his fingers. This he did regularly at his daily performances.

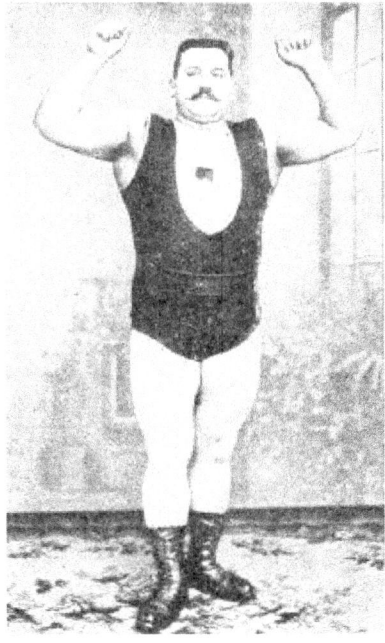

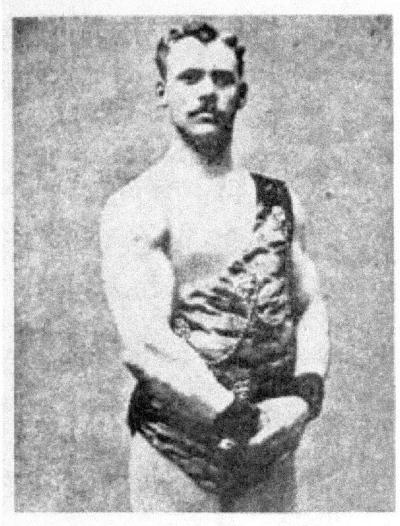

August Johnson, the great Swede who was recognized throughout Europe as the world's champion weight lifter. He was the only one who ever had the courage to challenge Cyr with a side stake. They met in Chicago in May, 1896, in the most memorable battle of strength in the world's history of strongmanism.

Louis Cyr as he was when he met Johnson, whom he said was the strongest man that he ever lifted against. On this occasion he shattered record after record in his rampage of strength. This photo gives you a good idea of the balanced proportions of his massive arms, which measured 19½ on the forearm and 22½ around the biceps. You would hardly think it, but he was the best-built "big man" that ever lived.

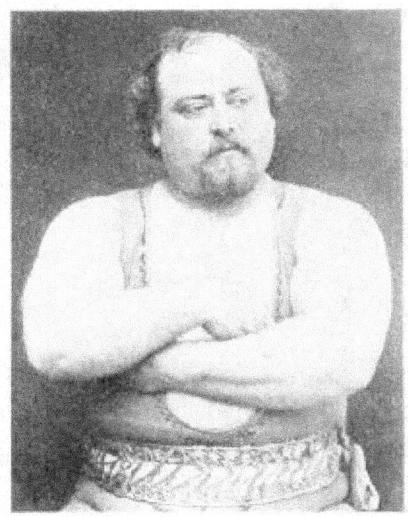

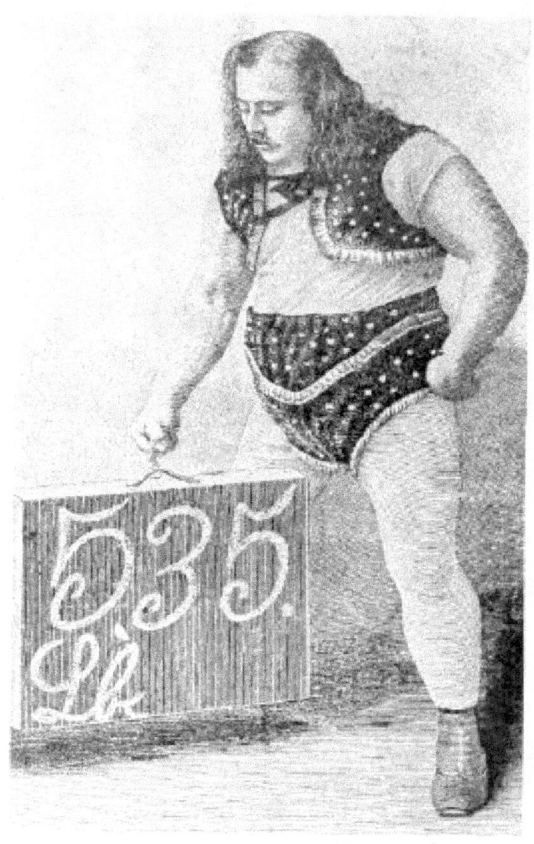

Cyr had finger strength in proportion to his great arm and body strength. His record finger lift was much higher than the marked poundage in the picture. It is claimed that in Chicago he raised 987 pounds with one hand and 1897½ pounds in the hand-and-thigh lift.

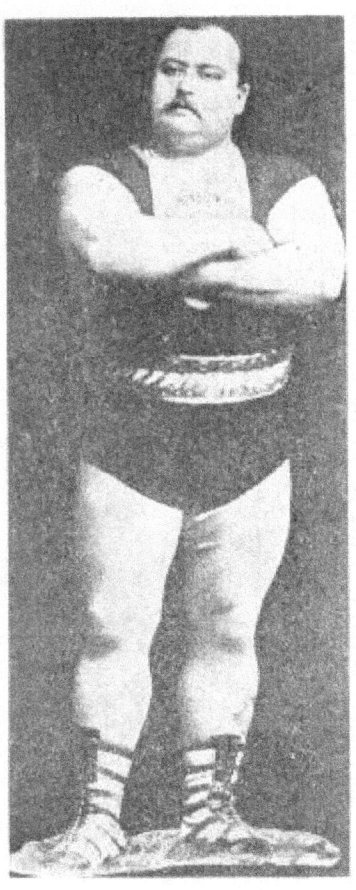

The great thunderbolt as he was when he crashed before the
British public on the night that he crushed Sandow's bent-press
record by pushing up with one hand over 273 pounds. Look how
clean-cut his legs are, and remember that his calf measured 28
inches, thigh 33 inches and over 50 inches around the hips. Then
you can better appreciate where his great body weight was and
why he remains "the strongest man that ever lived."

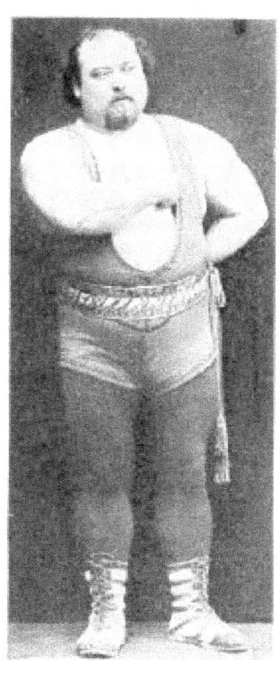

The arms and chest of Louis Cyr were so tremendous that Prof. Desbonnet said he never saw such enormous breadth of back, but his legs were majestically terrific. Impossible to describe. No wonder they are spoken of as props like the trunk of an oak. I fully believe, as so many who saw his great two-arm clean-and-jerk record of 347 pounds have told me, that it was more a press than anything else.

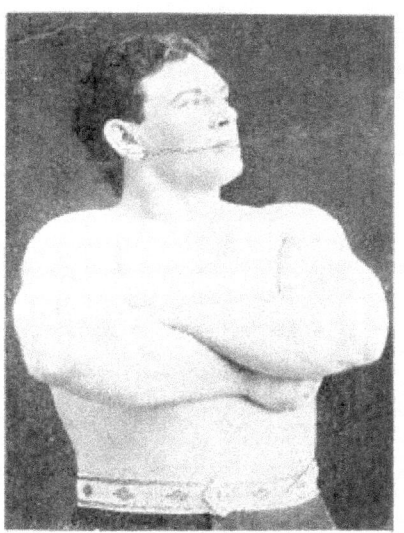

Hector DeCarrie, the young Montrealer upon whom Cyr bestowed his title in 1906, but did not transfer the belt, as DeCarrie failed to beat him.

15

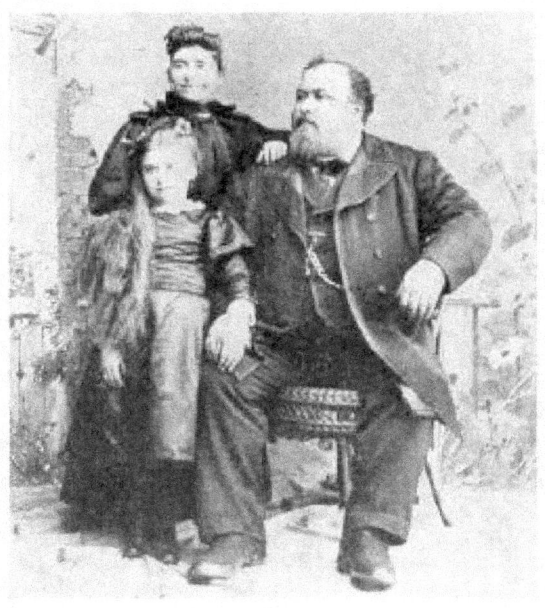

THE CYR FAMILY

The law of opposites—Madame Louis Cyr was as small as Louis was big, never weighing over 100 pounds. When Louis was in his prime he weighed around 315 pounds, all bone and muscle, a dynamo of power. By his side is his daughter, who gave a strong act with her father. The Mademoiselle married Dr. Ammou, of Montreal, where they both live and where also lives the aged mother, Madame Cyr.

his task as he straightened up to gaze into the dumfounded face of the speechless teamster. If the poor fellow had witnessed a miracle he could not have been any more astonished. With profuse thanks he climbed up into his wagon and drove off, his eyes filled with wonder and admiration. Later it was his delight to tell all with whom he came in contact of the doughty deed. In a country where the strength of a man is his deciding qualification, such news travels with incredible speed. The curiosity of the countryside was aroused, which brought a flow of callers to the Cyr home, under one pretext or another, in order to gaze upon the boy wonder. A crowd which never ceased until his death many years after.

Strength lovers were drawn toward him like moths to a flame, mostly to admire, although there were a few brave enough to cast doubt upon the extent of his bodily strength, but Louis suffered no doubting Thomases to remain long around him. They either put up or shut up. Nevertheless, the fact that he had become the center of attraction kindled apace the fires of his youthful enthusiasm and spurred him on to greater efforts. From the pastime of lifting logs and stones, he turned towards the implements of the professional strong man, and at the age of sixteen we find him daily contesting his strength against the records of others.

In the two years that intervened between the ages of sixteen and eighteen, his powers were only demonstrated locally, but the time was spent in building a solid rock for the fame that his future achievements were to bring him. So popular did he become that his name began to be spoken on equal terms with that of David Michaud, the reigning king of all Canadian strong men of that time; but the "fort l'homme" almost developed cholera to think that an eighteen-year-old boy should be considered his equal, let alone his superior. Just the same, popular opinion is as relentless as the tide which beats upon the shore, and day after day the shadow of the youthful Louis Cyr loomed greater and more insistently into his pathway.

In 1881 the inevitable happened for Michaud, and the match was made. They came together that same year and measured their strength against each other in Quebec, but not with bar bells or dumb bells as became the vogue later on in the French province. Rocks were the vehicles of resistance on this occassion, as they had always been with their Gaulish ancestors. The event became almost a national holiday. From out of the great south woods of Maine— once part of Quebec—came rugged men who prided themselves on the heftiness of their axe stroke, or their ability to wield a cant hook on a huge log, and their ability to run the logs downstream among the ice floes of springtime. Out of the north woods came the gaunt trappers and half-breed voyagers, who carried loads on the tump line over mountains and portages that would have crushed the ordinary man to the ground. East and west, from the farms, stores and business houses, men of all social grades, with but one thought in common, gathered to witness this struggle for supremacy between a boy in his 'teens and a seasoned giant of strength.

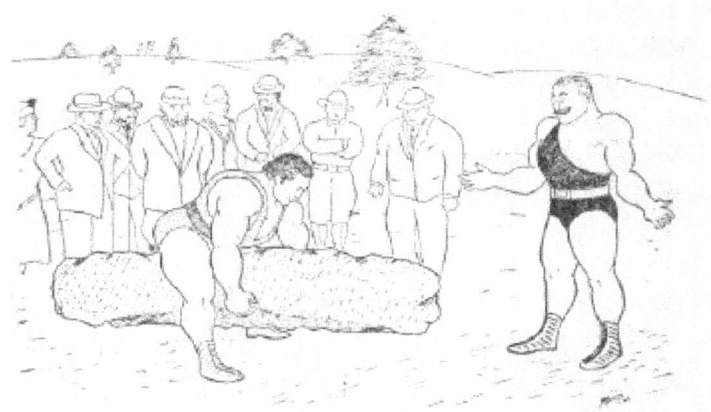

At the signal to commence Michaud stepped forward to his first task with the confident air of a man who knows his strength, and with no apparent exertion raised the awkward object from the ground—that was to be expected; but the interest was centered upon the youth whose turn came next. Quietly Louis moved from the circle of his friends and straddled the huge stone. Never for a moment did he pause as he placed his hands underneath the stone and tore it from the ground as easily as the champion did.

The multitude applauded vociferously as the St. Cyprien youth proved himself, causing interest to mount high. Michaud was astonished and muttered to himself, but manfully accepted the issue, and with a fixed determination he moved on towards the heavier stone. Again the champion was successful in raising the monstrous object from its setting, but there was a marked effort on his part this time. He took greater pains to set himself to balance the weight of the stone and clasp his hands under it. As he raised the stone the muscles of his back bulged, and the gnarled muscles on his arms and shoulders separated with the force of taxation. To some his legs seemed to tremble, and his regular breathing seemed to strangle into a tiny gasp— but it was a perfect lift and one that none of the spectators, but one, could duplicate. Louis stepped forward, a little pompously, as becomes a Frenchman, but there was that slight shadow of hesitancy within his eye that goes with youth and inexperience as it seeks to find its bearings. He paused at the stone, then walked around it. Satisfied with his observations, he stepped astride the stone and settled himself down to what had to be accomplished. The big form bulged and the neck shortened, and before the eyes of the tensed crowd the stone began to yield against a mightier resistance, so that once again the youthful challenger tied a lift with the champion Michaud.

All eyes now became centered upon a stone of greater size and awkwardness, which constituted the final test. Speculations ran high as to the ultimate outcome, and it is safe to say that the majority of the gathering placed their bets in favor of Cyr as the one of the two who would lift the stone, if it was to be lifted at all. It is impossible to describe the shape of this stone, as it had none, so to speak. As the time approached for Michaud to make his attempt it was plainly seen that an atmosphere of anxiety had formed among his followers. Michaud carried a look of uncertainty upon his face, and his step was less confident than before. However, he circled the boulder and rocked it several times in order to ascertain the axis of balance, and when he stepped astride his arms were taxed to circumnavigate it. Satisfied that he had secured the best grip possible, he bent his back to the task, pouring into his effort all his reserve —but not a move. His muscles twisted and writhed like live steel cables, and the veins in his throat stood out like whipcords. Still he fought it, and applied such great resistance that his feet were forced deep into the ground. Finally his fingers weakened and his hands slid away from their grip, leaving the stone as it was, unmoved. His bolt was shot; he stood aside, panting and trembling, a beaten man, with his gaze riveted upon the bulk of the youth who had now stepped forward to try his luck. From all sides a babble of advice poured upon young Louis in a jargon of confused, meaningless words, but he did not hear them, for he had his mind concentrated upon the issue that lay before him. His success in the second attempt and the apparent distress of the champion had given him great courage, and he stood astride the rock with less speculation than he had used before. His huge legs were set beneath him like the proverbial oak—props with which to conquer, and his massive back and arms glistened as the sun threw their waning rays upon his skin. As his arms spanned the stone, he breathed hard and commenced to lift; in response his young frame creaked under the terrific exertion. Time seemed to stand still and stretch into limitless space to the beholders who, with abated breath and riveted sight, hung upon each contracting muscle as he fought for supremacy.

A gasp went through the crowd as the stone was seen to move. They pressed forward as they saw it leave its bed, and broke into a roar of exultation as the young giant held it free from the ground. Daylight shone beneath it and the ground, as he held it suspended within his mighty arms several inches high. Here he paused a moment before he released his grip and then let the stone fall to the ground. With the characteristic display of the Frenchman, they hailed him with voice and gestures. Friends in thousands pressed around the eighteen-year-old Hercules to congratulate him as the new champion of Canada.

For many years this stone became a relic and a monument to his fame, and was revered by French Canadians with a fervor that was likened to that attributed to the stone of Jacob. The solid mass of stone was given out as having a weight of four hundred and eighty pounds. Some of you may be surprised to learn that stones of less weight than this had been used to tax the efforts of these two men of brawn. But did you ever weigh a large field stone? It is hardly likely that you have; otherwise you would not be surprised to find how much bulk is required to make up four hundred and eighty pounds. Some weigh much more than others, and granite for one exception is a great deal more compact and will considerably outweigh the average field stone of its dimensions. The stones used in this contest were of the boulder species, which are heavier than the general run of field stone. Generally they are very awkward, and their unwieldy bulk makes them terribly difficult to handle. The actual lifting of the stone depends upon its shape almost as much as its weight; and men have been known to exaggerate the weight of stones greatly, being misled by the bulk and awkwardness that cuts down the poundage they could lift under more favorable conditions.

At the age of eighteen Cyr was the symbol of strength in Canada, and he began to dream of other fields to conquer. His form had already reached Herculean proportions. The spread of his shoulders, twice the size of the ordinary strong man, concealed masses of muscle which lay in huge slabs upon their scaffold, and the depth and width of the pelvis was gigantic, even as the circumference of his powerful legs was beyond the belief of men who had never seen him.

The next three years found him persevering, and our next glimpse of him is caught on the eve of the year of his majority. At this time we find he had made a steady push, from the shoulder with one hand, of a dumb bell weighing two hundred and fifty pounds, and raised upon a platform with his back placed under it, a combined weight of iron and stone weighing two thousand nine hundred pounds. Slowly the news seeped through to other countries of this youthful Goliath, but no man believed it. Here in America we had Richard Pennell, who was looked upon as the greatest man of strength in the world. Seven years before Louis met the sturdy Michaud, Pennell had made the first one-arm record of any note at Wood's Gymnasium, in New York, by raising a dumb bell that weighed two hundred one pounds and four ounces. The world positively refused to believe that one so young as Louis had beaten that mark. Such disbelief almost thrust the great Louis down among the common herd, where he would have lived and died a hidden jewel of magnitude, but for the hand of fate.

During the year of 1885, Cyr went to Montreal to fulfill an engagement with Gus Lambert, a great patron of strong men, who then had a saloon in that ancient city. After concluding the engagement Louis decided to join the police force, since the prospect of making good as a strong man seemed to be very remote, due to the skeptical attitude of promoters and theatrical managers. It was just a temporary relapse, due to disappointment, that caused him to don the uniform at St. Gunegonde, a small village on the outskirts of Montreal. However, seven days after taking office, opportunity was to come to him in this secluded part of the world and hurl him before a startled public and so, eventually, launch him upon his great career. While on duty the seventh day, his march was arrested by the sound of profane altercation and the heavy thud of bodies colliding with each other. He paused a moment to locate the struggle, and with no further hesitation rushed to the scene where two burly men, much the worse for drink, were locked together in each others' arms, kicking, biting, gouging, and each trying his hardest to plunge a wicked-looking hunting knife into the other. Men fell back, afraid of the onslaught of the two powerful antagonists, but Louis plunged into them headlong and tore them apart, holding each of them at arm's length. Infuriated at being molested, they broke away and both turned upon Louis with murder in their eyes as they rushed upon him, knife in hand.

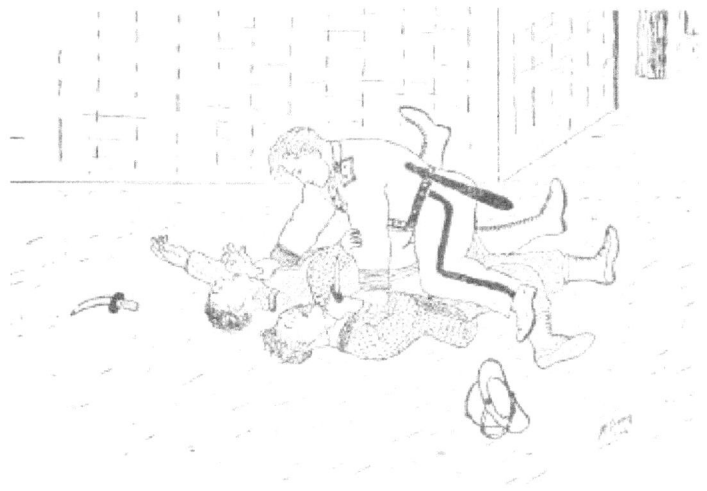

Little did they know what they were up against. Despite his huge bulk, Cyr was known throughout the province to be able to outfight and outwork any man as easily as he could outlift them. As the two men closed upon him, he grabbed each one by the breast of the shirt, which checked them with the same suddenness as if they had charged into a stone wall. Before they could recover the breath that had been knocked out of them, he had thrown them off their feet, face down in the dust of the road, with one huge, powerful knee rammed in the small of each back, pinning them down as securely as if they were spiked, while his hands tore the knives out of their hands and hurled them aside into the grass by the road. Badly hurt and exhausted from contact with this extraordinary human, they were unable to fight back, and their brains seemed to stand still as Cyr tucked one of them under each arm and walked to the police station in that manner, and dropped them in a heap before his amazed chief.

That night the Montreal papers were filled with the story, and the news spread all over the country like wildfire. It crossed the border into New York State and finally into the New York papers, where it drew the attention of Richard K. Fox, sportsman and publisher of "The Police Gazette," who was later to play a large part in the French Canadian's career.

I wonder if you have ever noticed the passion the French have for clean-cut logical sayings. If you have, you will, no doubt, recall the proverb which they have made very familiar and which is typical of the Gaulish mind. They say, "a door ought to be kept open or shut." This is a decided truism. Perhaps Louis believed in this proverb and decided it should be kept open for him so that he could step through when opportunity beckoned. The incident just related opened the door for him, and right then Louis definitely determined to become a professional performer. He resigned from the police force, but kept his saloon, which he had but recently opened. He threw out a defy to all and sundry to a contest, with the world's championship title as the issue and as much money as a side stake or wager as the other side cared to bet. He was now twenty-two years of age and began to fit out for himself an act with which to tour Canada and the United States. He stood five feet nine inches and weighed three hundred pounds, a mountain of iron, steel and stone, covered with straps and sheets of muscles as hard as rock. He was not a fat man as many imagine; his body was thick, almost square, built like a box. For so large a man he had an inspiring form. This is particularly true of his legs, which were very clean cut, despite their great size. Although there is no doubt about it that he was given to corpulency, it was not until later years that he showed it, when his weight went up to around four hundred pounds; but at this time he was living the years of enthusiasm, when his whole heart and soul were in his training and the testing of his daily increasing strength.

He liked to picture himself as the modern reproduction of the Biblical Samson, and his vision carried him on to the crest of the wave that was to sweep all opposition before him with the same all-conquering power as that of his ancient hero. No other man appealed to Louis as did that instrument of God, the son of Sarah.

He imitated his religious hero to the extent of wearing his hair in long tresses, which he wore cascading over his shoulders for many years. To him dumb bells and weight-lifting records of others were the Philistines—something to be conquered, and he attacked them with the same vigor as Samson of old fell upon his enemies. He was spectacular in a way beyond imitation and developed the inborn trait of the dramatic that belongs to the Latin mind; the skill that can provide a climax at a desired point when the beholders hang suspended upon the next movement, breathless, to be swept off their feet at the grand culmination.

In the year 1886, he met Richard Pennell for the premier strong-man honors of the world. On every feat he hopelessly outclassed the successor of Dr. Winship. Pennell was a finely built man and was looked upon as a wonder by reason of his great one-arm lift of two hundred and one pounds four ounces, which he performed at a body weight of one hundred and seventy-eight pounds, when he was twenty-eight years of age. He was in his fortieth year when he clashed with Cyr, who was then in his twenty-third year. The record made by Pennell is the first bent press on record, and he is credited as being the originator of this lift, but I think the honors are divided. Louis Attila, the European strong man, was the first to develop the lift in Europe, and he later taught it to Eugene Sandow, who made it so popular; but there is no doubt in my mind that Pennell thought the lift out himself, as this was many years before Attila or any of the formidable Europeans came to America. Neither one knew of the other, yet the American's record was greater than Attila's at that time.

Matches in those dawning days of strongman- ism were not conducted as are the matches of today. Each man selected a set of his own pet lifts, and each had to follow the other through his routine. The man who did better on the other man's set of lifts was adjudged the winner. He did not always have to outlift his opponent; that was to be decided by the judges, and some weird decisions were handed out, as was proven by the Sandow-McCann match and the Sandow- Saxon lift.

The followers of Pennell smiled as they saw Cyr go through his set of back lifts, finger lifts and other dead lifts that were raised just off the floor, followed by his manipulation of barrels of sand. They figured Cyr was built for those stunts, and Pennell would do better in the judge's eyes than Cyr would on Pennell's lifts. They believed that the Pennsylvania University instructor would tie the huge man up in what they termed arm lifts. They were to learn that the bulk of the French Canadian's arms was muscle and not fat. As Pennell made his one- arm press of two hundred pounds, he wore a satisfied smile, but it soon faded and he became dumfounded to see Cyr pick the same weight up as though it was a bag of peanuts and shove overhead with no perceptible body bend. His next lift was a revelation as Cyr rolled forward a huge dumb bell. People speculated on the weight of the dumb bell, many scoffing and saying it was hollow; but this was just one of Louis' ideas to create an effect. He tossed the bell to the shoulder, and stiff-legged, with a limited body bend, he slowly thrust the weight to arms' length. Letting it crash to the floor, he calmly said, "Weigh it." Curiosity became amazement as the announcer cried out, "Two hundred and fifty-three pounds." Reporters and sportsmen alike began to realize that there was foundation to the news that had drifted across the St. Lawrence to their ears, and before the contest was over they were satisfied that they were looking upon the man who comes only once in so many hundred years, according to some statisticians.

Pennell was great in a one-arm curl and often curled one hundred pounds. During this contest he curled one hundred and two pounds, but the lift faded into insignificance as the youthful Cyr curled twenty-five pounds more. Pennell did not have a chance on a single lift; thus Louis Cyr became recognized all over the American Continent as the strongest man in the world. He had nothing else but honest praise for the man he beat, and Louis came to respect the man who has been given credit for starting the strong-man movement in America as well as being instrumental in forwarding physical exercise as an educational feature in the schools. Pennell was connected with Dr. Sargeant and, among many others, Dr. Winship. Dr. Flint, of New York, the man who won fame as alienist in the Harry Thaw-Stanford White case, was an excellent pupil of Richard Pennell. He was an unusually powerful man^ being capable at any time of pressing his own weight with either hand, which stood at one hundred and eighty pounds. We are indebted to Pennell for this pupil, who was the father of Dr. Flint, Jr., the man who wrote an interesting, instructive volume on exercise, which at that time was a masterpiece.

As so very little is known of Pennell, I feel sure that you will not object if I leave the French-Canadian monarch for a while to tell you a story in which Richard was proven the unexpected master. He was born in America in 1846, although many have stated he was an Englishman, but that was only by extraction. Fully dressed, he was not an inspiring man; only when stripped he did look the part. His best lifting weight was one hundred and seventy- eight pounds, and as a young man he joined the circus of Batchellor and Doris, daily exhibiting his strength. When they were showing in Syracuse, N. Y., a rube came up to him after the performance with more of his friends who had come in to see the circus. Tapping Pennell on the chest, the rube remarked, "Well, you may be a strong man, but we have a man who can beat you on pitching quoits the furthest."

"That may be," replied Pennell, "for I have never thrown quoits, but I doubt it very much."

"Well, we've got fifty bucks to say he is a better man at his distance," the rube came back, and just as promptly he pulled out a wad of greenbacks and began to thumb off fifty. Just as promptly Dick pulled out his fifty and said, "I bet that your man can't meet me at my distance." The stakes put up, the rube asked, "What is your distance?"

"Never mind," Pennell reiterated. "Stick up your peg on your man's distance, and I'll show you."

One hundred and fifty feet were stepped off and a stake driven into the ground to mark it. The champion rube pitcher stepped up, coat off, shirt sleeves rolled up, and throat bared, to do his stuff. Right on the one hundred and fifty mark his quoit landed, and a tickled sensation trilled through the bunch of rural sports. It was a husky throw, indeed, for the quoits used were considerably heavier than those pitched today. "Ha, Ha, so that's it," Dick said, and stooped to pick up a quoit without unbuttoning his coat. He toed the line, eyed the distance and then stepped back, and "whang," the quoit sailed through the air, landing fully twenty feet past the mark of the rube. "That's my mark," Dick grinned, as he coolly collected his own fifty and the rube's fifty and walked away from the gaping throng.

Pennell was enormously strong, as judged by the times; and at wrist-turning and curling weights he was considered invincible until he met his Waterloo in Louis Cyr. In a match with Henry Holtgrewe, the Cincinnati strong man, on wrist-turning and curling weights, which were Henry's specialty, Pennell won in a decisive manner, irrespective of Holtgrewe's body weight advantage; but either of these two men might just as vainly have tried to turn over a house single-handed as to have tried to budge the arm of Cyr a fraction of an inch.

# CHAPTER II

After showing his superiority over Pennell, Cyr continued with his show throughout the New England States. After appearing in Boston, he went to Lawrence, Massachusetts, where he showed for one night. It was at about this time that our old friend Oscar Matthes, who lived in Lawrence, was at his best. Louis had heard a lot of talk about Oscar, and on the morning following his professional appearance, he and his manager called upon the little fellow. They were joyfully received, and although Louis at this time was three times the size of Oscar, yet each was as big-hearted as the other and as wrapped up in their pet sport of lifting weights. In honor of the visit, Oscar did some lifting which greatly astonished the big man. He could hardly believe a man of one hundred and nine pounds could lift so much weight, but then Matthes was as great a king in his class as Louis was in his. Unfortunately, Oscar did not have all of his weights on hand and was obliged to tie small weights on an eighty-pound bar bell in order to make his lifts. At the conclusion Louis took a fifty-pound thick-handled dumb bell and crossed it over the center of the eighty-pound bar bell, and with no exertion at all curled them in this awkward manner, using only one hand, and pressed the combined weights to alms' length many times. While he remained fully dressed, he next laid his friend, a man of one hundred and eighty pounds, on the palm of one hand and pressed him to arms' length. Oscar said Louis looked like a real apostle of might, with his long-flowing hair and gigantic form. Louis was so big that he had to travel sideways through the door and along the corridor, and then he almost required a shoe horn to help him through the more narrow inner house doors. Not a chair in the house was large enough for him to place his huge bulk upon, and this obliged him to be seated upon the couch, which groaned under the bur den of his weight with every movement. The Matthes found Louis and his manager very courteous, and Cyr not given to speak much of himself. He was still in his twenty-third year and weighed three hundred and fifteen pounds on his visit to the miniature Hercules. The following two years saw his time divided, showing at various places and at his saloon in Montreal, where he delighted his patrons, and especially the draymen, at the way he juggled around the barrels of beer, which weighed around three hundred pounds.

It was in the year of 1888, on October 1st, at Berthierville, Quebec, that he again aroused public interest with a great back-lift, raising a platform off all four corners. It was loaded down with pig iron totaling three thousand five hundred and thirty-six pounds. This was the first great record that he nailed to his mast, and a proof that his limitations were far from being reached, as the succeeding years testified. Cyr varied his lifting, including dumb-bell and barbell work with back lifts, dead lifts, and fingerlifts.

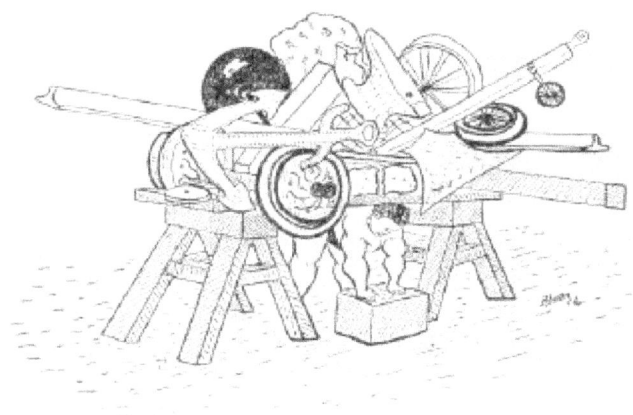

Of the whole set of lifts, dumb bells took precedence in overhead lifting. Even when two hands were employed, two dumb bells were selected in preference to a bar bell. I can quite understand why Louis preferred dumb bells in the place of bar bells, simply because his great bulk made him better able to pick up separate dumb bells than the bar bell. The way he would get the dumb bell to his shoulders was to lift one up as far as the waist so that it rested on the thick part of his thighs; then he stooped over and pulled the other up likewise. From this position it was no trouble at all for him to get them to his shoulder and raise them overhead. His hardest task was to raise them off the floor. The average lifter would find it an enormous task to raise two dumb bells from the thigh to the shoulder, as the back bend required for leverage is great and also dangerous—but not so with Cyr. His great bulk had fashioned his back like the trunk of a great tree—unbendable, and the depth of muscle flanking the spine was almost incredible. Naturally, his back became a pry of terrific power. There was no hol- low in the small of the back, which is so often seen in the average person—his back could retain its rigidity under great resistance. The most singular thing to me is why French Canadian athletes retain the affection for separate dumb bell lifting, even up to the present time. They are more awkward to handle than a bar bell and require greater effort to raise overhead. Probably it is this practice which makes them so efficient when they come to handle bar bells, which it later did for Cyr.

1889 saw him performing at St. Henri, Quebec, when he made his second record and first overhead record, shoving a dumb bell weighing two hundred and sixty-five pounds to arms' length. A few years afterwards, Eugene Sandow laid his claim to the world's championship by breaking this record with four pounds. How great the imagination of some people is. Great as Sandow was in his line, he was a pigmy alongside of the great Louis, and to stop and compare their respective powers would be a joke, more than a waste of time. Sandow performed his record with a dumb bell placed on a block of wood six inches high; he then rocked it to the shoulder, using both hands, and raised it to arms' length in what was termed in those days "a screw lift." Years ago its name was changed to the "bent press." Cyr could no more bent press than fly. His great legs never bent at the knees, and I very much doubt if he bent over sideways any more than six inches. The width of the small of his back and the depth of his pelvis would not permit it. Louis stood the dumb bell on end, resting the other end against his thigh, and by prying with one hand he pulled the weight over to the shoulder and pushed to arms' length. Such a feat was a sheer impossibility for Sandow to attempt, let alone duplicate. The enormous legs of the Montrealer were the secret of his strength. They were the sustaining props of power that could resist a greater pressure than the bulwark of might that reared above them could handle. The world has never since produced a man with legs the size of Cyr's. Try and imagine a thirty-three inch thigh and twenty-eight inch calf! That is what he had, and if there was one part of his body that was clean-cut and beautiful to look at, it was those terrific legs. The knee and the calf and ankle were perfectly moulded. Up to his last days they retained their magnificent shapeliness. It was these supernormally developed underpinnings that considerably composed his body weight. People who never saw him did not take the possibility of such legs into consideration, which caused many, even athletes, to believe that Louis Cyr was just a monstrosity of flesh. He was to be a revelation to everybody. I can safely say that he was the best- proportioned man of his weight who ever lived. His best measurements after reaching maturity were: height, 5 feet 10¼ inches; weight, stripped, 295 pounds; normal chest, 59½ inches; waist, 47 inches; biceps, 22½ inches; forearm, 19½ inches; thigh, 33 inches; calf, 28 inches. Of course, you will perfectly understand that a man with such huge proportions could not be expected to have exactly what we would call a graceful figure. As I once laughingly but truly told a friend, "Cyr was built for service, not beauty." Still you do not see the huge bulging abdomen as expected of a man of his weight There is a difference of twelve and one-half inches between his chest and waist, and we could not expect nature to give a smaller waist measurement and retain the powerful construction to balance with such sized legs which formed hips of over fifty-inch circumference. His flesh was hard as stone, and you could not make a dent into his flexed biceps or legs. If anything, his neck was a little too short, but overlooking that point, he was pretty well proportionate. His forearm measurement exceeded that of Apollon, the Parisian giant, whose arm has been said to be the largest measured of any strong man. The Frenchman of new France was infinitely more powerful in proportion to his greater measurements than the idol of old France. Stanislaus Zbyszko claimed to have the largest circumference of upper arm, and indeed had tremendous triceps, but he lacked half an inch of equaling the biceps of Louis, and was a million miles behind as far as strength was concerned. Despite the extraordinary immensity of his proportions, this leviathan had a majesty of carriage all his own, which, as I previously have written, was never imitated by any strong man of his time or any who came after. Dr. Sargeant marveled at Cyr and said, after a physical examination, that Louis was as hard as mahogany.

Louis' great fault was eating. He was a genuine gourmand, and in his stages of inactivity between matches and show performances, he increased his weight enormously, and more so in the later years of his life when contentment came with conquest. The lightest body weight he ever made was in 1896, when he contested against August Johnson in Chicago. He then weighed two hundred and seventy pounds, but his general lifting body weight was around three hundred and fifteen pounds.

The year following his record performance at St. Henri, we find him in another record- creating frame of mind, which was celebrated on the night of November 21, 1890. No less than twenty-seven times was counted as he pressed a solid dumb bell of one hundred and nine pounds to arms' length in a series of repetition lifts. Fourteen days later, on December 5th, he made a one-finger lift, raising a solid mass of iron weighing four hundred and ninety pounds off the floor, using the middle finger only. These feats were sufficient with which to greet the approaching Christmastide and wind up the old year. Then dawned the year of 1891, the epoch-making year in the annals of strengthdom, which brought together from all parts of the universe rivals of immeasurable quality who were to meet and write their names indelibly upon the sands of time. The whole world was aroused, and the multitudes that turned out to see the struggles for physical conquest and pay homage to the conqueror were greater than has ever been assembled since in the sport of heavy weight lifting. For several years the passion to witness feats of strength continued. These were the feast years for the sons of Hercules, Titan, Vulcan, Anak, Atlas and Samson, and around their heroic forms and deeds romance has wrapped a cloak of enthralling magic which stirs within the most conventional breast a longing to be a man among men. These years caused the primitive seeds of Adam to struggle to the surface for a little while to remind many of us of our utter inefficiency, but, nevertheless, kindled the idealism within us to admire and deify the man that God made.

England was in the throes of another Gothic invasion, which swept over the sea-girt isle in a flood of conquest that outrivaled the invasion of their Anglo-Saxon ancestors. This was a conquest of the heart made by the heroic forms of mighty men who did more than any statesman to help Victorian England throw off the shackles of false pride and prudery, to which she was enslaved. Among the first were Sampson and Cyclops and the McCann brothers, who were astounding the British public with their remarkable demonstrations of strength. Later came the meteor Sandow, who shook England like an earthquake, creating an enthusiasm that paved the way for the thunderbolt Cyr, who was to crash among them and stun them with his superior feats; capping the climax created by the great forerunners.

The first to arrive in America was Sebastian Miller, a huge German, reputed to be possessed of extraordinary strength. So well satisfied was he of his own abilities being superior to Cyr, that he eagerly plunged into a match with the long-haired giant, who, since he had defeated all on the American continent, welcomed the opportunity to pit his strength against a foreigner of renown. They signed the agreement to meet on the evening of July 2nd in Montreal. Nowadays, when an athlete signs a contract for a match of any kind, he forgets everything else and trains industriously upon the issue in question. Everything is done to husband his strength, and if he was asked to perform during that time he would think the one who asked such a request was crazy to harbor such a thought. This was not the fact in Louis' days. Four days before the scheduled match, Cyr gave an exhibition, going his limit on many of his feats. In one of his stunts he excelled any previous performance. Grasping a barrel of cement by the chines, using only one hand, he rocked it on the thigh, and from there up on his shoulder and then walked away with it. The barrel weighed three hundred and fourteen pounds, a feat which always stuck his opponents. It is strange that Cyr could be so efficient in barrel stunts, as one would naturally expect his great size to interfere with handling such unwieldy objects. They were generally filled with cement, sand or a mixture of sand and water, but they did not bother him, as may be judged from the great poundages he handled.

The night of the match Louis was feeling splendidly buoyed with enthusiasm for testing his mettle against the husky Teuton. But the result was the same as in his other contests. Miller was hopelessly outclassed. The honor of first lift was given to the visitor, who raised a bar bell weighing two hundred and thirty-two and one-half pounds overhead with two hands in a press lift. The first move our Louis did caused the confidence of the German to evaporate. The Big Canadian strode forward and almost took the weight out of Miller's hand, as he laid it on the floor and took it to the shoulder in one movement, using the overhand grip, as used in the one-hand snatch. Receiving the weight at the shoulder, he spun it around, ducking his head so that the weight could be better handled at the shoulder. To the consternation of all, Louis pushed the weight up four times in succession with the right arm. Miller next tried a back lift and quit at two thousand four hundred pounds, a low poundage for the sized man he was. Cyr did not stop lifting until he had raised three thousand one hundred and ninety-two pounds, which at that was way below his best. As he later said, he saw he had the German easily outclassed and had no desire to beat him too badly. Cyr next duplicated his barrel feat of three hundred and fourteen pounds, which he had lifted four nights before, but, according to the newspaper reports of that match, Cyr was explained as placing the barrel on the shoulder with one hand and without the use of his legs. By that they meant that Cyr did not pull the barrel on the thigh and rest it there before it was shouldered. He might have laid the barrel on its side and placed the buckle of his big belt under the top part of the chine, and then by reaching over with the hand grasp the chine at the further end of the barrel and by pulling over use the belt buckle as a base in place of the knee. They used to lift a heavy dumb bell to the shoulder by allowing the large nut at one end to catch on the belt. However, Miller could not do anything with the barrel. They passed on to the stone-breaking contest, which Miller won, as he also won the next feat of lifting a heavy barrel of sand off the floor by grasping it by the chines with both hands. It is a cinch that Cyr let Miller get away with that lift, and Miller knew it.

In my home town there was an old sportsman who was a conductor on the Canadian Railroad. He told me that by accident he found himself sitting opposite Miller while eating in a restaurant the day of this match. Naturally Mr. Johnson began to ask Miller his chances. He told me that Miller laughed out loud as he told him that he would be an easy winner. He said, "Cyr is so big that he cannot bend over, so how can he lift big weights?" Miller and Mr. Johnson met again in the same restaurant the next day when slyly Mr. Johnson remarked, "I thought that you were going to win?" Miller shook his head as he replied, "I never thought it possible for him to lift so much, and he did it all so easily." In other words, Miller knew that Cyr was lifting well within himself. It might interest some of my readers to know that Sebastian Miller settled down in America, and his son is "Hack" Miller, the famous baseball player, generally spoken of as the "strong man of baseball."

# CHAPTER III

Louis Cyr was elated over his new victory, while the newspapers ran huge front-page headlines and columns of write-ups on the popular idol. Feeling that his title was really established, Cyr availed himself of his increased popularity and set out again for the New England States with his show. He was not to remain long, for unknown to him some of the chief figures in the British invasion from Europe were transferring their scene of activity to the American side of the Atlantic Ocean. Cyclops, to whom I made a passing reference as being one of the main actors in the activities in England with Sampson, had split with his partner. In fact they had not gotten along so well since the night that Eugene Sandow, with his friend and advisor, Louis Attila, had invaded the platform when the Cyclops-Sampson act came on, and wrecked the show. This was in 1889. To add more coals to the fire, the popularity afforded Sandow had caused their sun to diminish. Then it was that the pupil of Sampson broke away and came in contact with Montgomery Irving, an Englishman, who had a fine physique, not unlike that of Sandow and was morever very good looking. Between them they conspired, and Cyclops hit the bright idea of getting even with Sandow, the man who had caused all his trouble, by setting out for America in company with Irving under the heading of "Cyclops and San- dowe, The World's Strongest Men." You will notice that the name "Sandowe" was spelled with an "e" on the end. Masquerading as the real Sandow and relying upon being accepted as such, the two men arrived in New York with their act in 1891, a few days after the Miller- Cyr contest. Hearing that Cyr had left Montreal on tour, they decided to locate there and take the opportunity provided by his absence, and clean up. At the very beginning, their ill- founded plans were to react upon them and tumble around their ears in disaster in a sensational manner. It is regretted, as they were both very capable men. Cyclops was extremely strong and was reputed to have the strongest hands of any man in the world. His right name was Franz Bienkowski, the son of a Dantzig blacksmith, who built up his reputation on his remarkable ability to break coins with his fingers. Many people do not believe that this is possible, and many students of strength disbelieve that any human being can thus break a coin into halves. I suppose because men whom they have known to be accredited with such finger strength were not able to do the feat when put to the test. Yet there have been such men capable of taking a coin between the fingers and breaking it through the center. I have witnessed the feat done twice during my lifetime, and I can quite understand the reason for disbelief, as men of that calibre are rare. Bienkowski, or Cyclops I should better call him, was one of them. On one occasion when he was appearing at Lille, in France, he was challenged by one of the audience to break his coin, which Cyclops did.

The story of this came to the ears of an athlete named Noel, who was an instructor in a gymnasium, at Boulets, where Cyclops was booked to appear. As soon as he arrived, Noel with many other French strong men went to him and to his face accused him of being a faker. Noel worked himself up into a rage, finally challenging, "Here is a coin you will not break so easily as the one you broke up North. Let us see if you can, and 100 francs if you do it." Cyclops, with a grin, took the franc, which is about the size of a quarter, and with no great effort broke it before their eyes. "Give me another," Cyclops said, and with a few twists broke it. "And another, and another," he cried, and so took them from the hands of Noel and his friends until he had broken a dozen. "Now give me the 100 francs," he said.

Cyclops performed this feat before Professors Bonnes and Desbonnet, of France, and alongside of the coins broken by Vanstittart and Marx in the French strong-man museum lays a coin broken by Cyclops. Despite his great finger strength, Desbonnet did not have a high regard for the lifting records of Cyclops. When Professor Desbonnet recited the broken-coin feat in "La Culture Physique," the professor said, "Cyclops claims to have military pressed a two- hundred-pound bar bell seven times in succession." To this he injected the little phrase of sarcasm, "Incorrectly, of course." A Frenchman has no regard for a German. Somehow I always get a great kick out of a Frenchman's version of a German athlete, and vice versa. I have a mean weakness to draw comment from one about the other whenever I have the pleasure of meeting a good French or German strong man.

Only one man was ever proven the master of Cyclops in breaking coins, and that was the big, happy-souled John (Gruhn) Marx. Cyclops could neither bend the same sized horseshoe nor break the same coins that Marx could. Professor Paulinetti had a dime that John broke for him, which is the smallest sized coin I ever heard of being broken. The fact that it is so small makes the feat more difficult. But an American quarter, Bah! He would hold it in front of your face and count "one, two, three, four," and the thing was broken.

There I go again. Whenever I get telling of strong-man feats, my mind becomes filled with comparisons. Just as my soul becomes saturated with the whole subject, then I am apt to wander. So I will get back to our gigantic friend by saying such was the man who arrived in Montreal, the summer of 'ninety-one with Montgomery Irving, whose name has gone down in strongman annals as "The false Sandow."

Cyr was in Worcester, Massachusetts, when he received a wire announcing the presence of these two men in Montreal. Friends of Louis were angered at the broad, sweeping challenges the invaders were hurling in every direction. "Where is this man Cyr?" they cried. "If he is so good, why does he run away when he knows we are here?

Bring him forth, and Cyclops, the conqueror of the world, will break him as easily as he breaks this coin." Their ravings and wild statements drew immense crowds, and the people on every hand called out for Cyr. The telegram urged Louis to return immediately, and without a moment's loss of time. The idol of America broke up his show and took the first train bound for Montreal. A great crowd of friends were on hand to welcome him as the train drew into Bonaventure Station. Into his ears they poured the facts, their fancies and impressions of the two imposters until Louis was filled with an honest, just rage. Cyclops might be strong— the coin-breaking stuff had created a great impression over everyone—but he, Louis Cyr, would sweep him off his pedestal as the sea carries a rock away from a sandy base. Radio could not have broadcast Louis' homecoming more rapidly. The city just seethed with excitement, and, strange as it may seem, the bombastic two did not know of Cyr's arrival until he filled the aisle with his huge bulk, a threatening Nemesis.

As the time neared for the theatre doors to open, a mob of excited, milling humanity besieged the box office. An orderly line-up was out of question, as the police were powerless to control the disorderly mob. The showmen and their manager reckoned the crowd in a different light. To them it was the result of their ability and showmanship. They speculated on the golden harvest that was before them, which made them heady; so they opened the show that night more brazenly than ever. Every seat was taken and the aisles were crowded, while the balcony creaked under the load that it held. Every act was panned, as yells, shrieks and cat calls in French and English tore the air with ear-splitting static for the men of brawn. Finally the curtain rang up on the strong-man show to reveal a display of weights of monstrous proportions, besides other apparatus used for various stunts. As the false Sandowe and the huge Cyclops took up their positions on either side of the stage amid its herculean scenery, Mr. King, their manager, advanced to the footlights, holding high his hands besieging silence from a multitude of people who apparently had lost all control of their vocal chords. All that was heard were shouts of "Cyclops," "Cyr," which rose and fell in waves as the crowd felt the exertion of their continued shouting, or broke in as they regained their wind. At last they began to realize that all the noise was getting them nothing and gradually subsided into silence. King began to talk. He spoke of the great success of Sandowe in England—stealing the real Sandow honors and giving the crowd the idea that the Sandow who stormed England was the same man who stood before them. He extolled the physical beauty of Irving, which was to a certain extent justified, and might have brought Irving great success if he had been genuine with himself. Then King turned to describe the further wonders of Cyclops; he—well, what is the use of boring you with the mass of lies that King fabricated. That man could lie faster than a dog could trot, but the moment he began to decry Cyr a threatening murmur arose from the crowd. Their vindication of a great man was not necessary, for, as the words of denunciation hung upon the lips of the crowd a ponderous figure cast its shadow down the aisle. As the form advanced, people craned their necks, and the syllable, "Cyr," was framed in every mouth, to be hurled from wall to wall in a deafening bombardment. Men left their seats and women forgot their deportment as they stood upon the chairs to catch a glimpse of the man who was sternly marching down the aisle toward the stage to defend his name and honor. The almost maniacal roar of the multitude which now issued struck the imposters with deadening force, from which they recoiled as the deafening word of "Cyr, Cyr," throbbed into their brain with the sickening thud of a doom bell.

Cyr heard nothing, saw nobody from the moment he flung open the door but the three forms that stood upon the stage, the men who had flaunted his name with their cowardly recriminations. His eyes focused upon the face of Cyclops, he marched down between the cheering people, closely followed by his manager, Mr. Labadie, and another; Louis clambered on the stage, completely ignoring the Teuton's manager as he strode up to the big German, whose form seemed to shrink as the shadow of the avenger loomed upon him. Only the hulk of Cyr's body, which completely obliterated the other from view, prevented the clamoring audience from realizing the startled effect produced upon Cyclops. He was frozen in amazement by the gigantic form of the man before him, and his tongue seemed to cleave to the roof of his mouth, refusing to respond to the few remaining sparks of intelligence that struggled through his paralyzed brain.

Deep, burning anger smouldered in the big, honest eyes of Louis, as he demanded of Cyclops, "You say that I run away from you— that I will not pit my strength against your strength, because I am afraid. Produce your feats and I will beat them. Do not think, M'sier, because you break a few coins between your fingers that you can make us believe you are the strongest man in the world. You must beat me first." With these words tumbling from his lips, Louis pitched his coat, collar and vest into the stage wings, sufficiently attired and ready to meet the boaster on his own ground.

Things were progressing differently between the respective managers; each was voluble, but Mr. King was getting the worst of it. In the delirium of words that surged around him, he felt like a cockleshell buffeted from wave to wave in a mid-Atlantic storm. Helplessly he turned to his partners, but they were just as much at sea. Labadie was demanding immediate action. "We are here to accept your double challenge in which you offer $500.00 to the man who defeats SanJowe, and $1000.00 to the man who can duplicate all of Cyclops' feats. "I have the men here," he cried, waving his hand in the direction of his two companions. King tried to spar for time. This was too sudden. He begged for another night, but Labadie was obdurate. "You throw your mud and think you will get away with it, but you won't," he stormed. "None of you will leave this theatre tonight without proving your men can beat mine, or my men can beat yours."

Seeing there was no other way out, and fearing lest they become the victims of the maddened crowd, he advised Cyclops and Irving to do what they could. Thus the dual match commenced.

Louis followed Cyclops on feat after feat, which all were of a minor order according to the strength of the Montrealer. All the time the spectators kept up a storm of raillery mixed with cheers and banter; and throughout it all, shouts called continually for "the big bell," "the big bell," alluding to an enormous-sized dumb bell which Cyclops lifted nightly, with claims that no man in the world but himself could raise it from the shoulder to arms' length. His story was that he had traveled the world and every man who tried to lift it had failed. There is no disputing the fact that this lift was good. The bell weighed two hundred and fifty pounds and had a very awkward handle. I was told on several occasions that many athletes of genuine good standing could not get it even to the shoulder. Therefore, I can readily believe that Cyclops had greater confidence in himself on this feat for the final coup and hoped to show Cyr up accordingly. In response to the demands of the people, he ordered the big bell rolled forward. With a dramatic gesture he grasped the dumb bell by the handle, and with a heave supplied with both hands he got it to the shoulder. Pressing and bending over sideways to an acute angle, he raised the weight to arms' length. The audience applauded, for they recognized a hefty lift, and they were eager to see how Louis would make out, as every one there had not seen him perform his previous record. Louis was out for blood this night, if ever he was, and was as willing as the crowd was eager for him to come to grips with the mass of iron. To the shoulder it came, and with hardly any perceptible bend he thrust the weight upward on its arm-length journey. Every one did three things at once—they stamped, clapped and whooped in a crescendo of noise enough to waken the dead. Cyclops was amazed, as most people are at seeing their stuff duplicated; but he and his manager rushed forward into an argument, accusing Louis of not performing the lift correctly. Labadie nearly developed an apoplectic fit, while the favorite spread his arms wide in indignation as his brows raised with surprise. Meanwhile, the crowd added their stanza of disgust, emphasized by groans and cat calls. "What," Louis exploded, "I did not lift the dumb bell right! Why I lifted it easier than he does," he added with an accusing finger. "To prove it I will do it again," and to the surprise of every one, including Cyclops, Louis grabbed the weight a second time, and in his rage he pulled the weight to the shoulder in a single movement; and with eyes staring upon his accuser he pressed the weight aloft, as he roared, "Does that satisfy you," pointing with the other hand to the ascending weight. Aloft he held it, as he stood with feet wide apart, legs rigid as steel pillars, until Cyclops nodded his head in satisfaction, signifying the lift was a better one than his own. A pandemonium of glee followed, which lasted into the early hours of the morning, as the idol worshippers drank themselves recklessly drunk, toasting their hero.

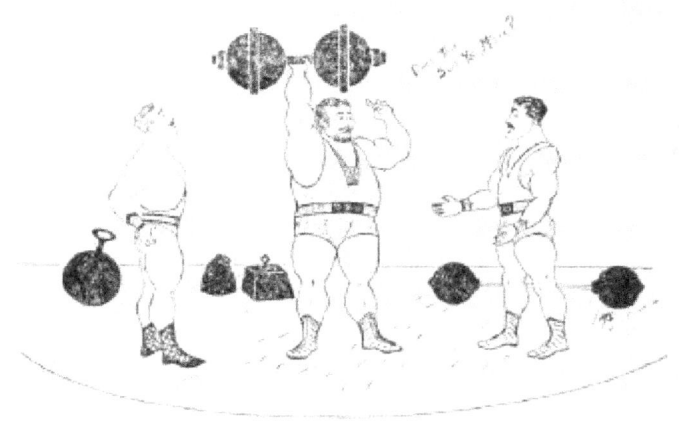

Montgomery Irving was also easily defeated by the youthful pupil of Louis Cyr, who was none other than Horace Barre. Louis discovered this young giant in his native province when Barre was only a boy. He later referred to him as "the boy still in his teens" whom he was taking to London to beat the real Sandow, where he would show the inhabitants of the tight little isle what real strength was. The arrival of Cyclops and Sandowe provided the chance for Louis to test his protege, but Irving's best lifts were not enough to make Horace feel warm. Naturally, they were a much-elated pair that night on their success in calling the boasters' bluff, but even at that Louis was not satisfied. Deep down in his heart was a thirst to teach the wilful braggarts a lesson. Why should men like them be allowed to besmirch the names and abilities of men who were good and loved the profession and followed it honorably. Louis realized that all he had done was to show to the public that the weights of Cyclops could be lifted, but Cyclops had not proven that he could do any one stunt that he, Louis Cyr, could do. Consequently, he reasoned how was the public to know he was a much better man than Cyclops. Thoughts began to become realities as the three got their heads together and decided to invade the "Cyclops-Sandowe" show the next night. Wednesday night arrived and the theatre doors opened, admitting three men among the regular audience who took their seats in the first row to impatiently await the feature act of the night. As the curtain rose announcing the strong-man turn, Mr. Labadie leaped upon the stage before Mr. King could say a word. He held up his hand and began to address the audience. "Ladies and gentlemen, last evening you will readily recall how our great citizen, Louis Cyr, the only man in the world entitled to call himself the world's strongest man, met Cyclops on Mr. King's terms and successfully demonstrated his ability to do everything that Cyclops did. The manner in which Louis Cyr did those lifts proved that he is a much stronger man than Cyclops, and we are here tonight to prove to you beyond a shadow of doubt that our citizen is the strongest man in the world. Last night Cyr lifted every weight Cyclops did, and now in all fairness we ask Cyclops to lift the weights that Cyr will lift. We have brought our weights with us and a wager of $1000.00 that Cyclops cannot follow Cyr half-way through his set of lifts. I might further say that the money of fered by Cyclops and Sandowe to anyone who successfully beat them according to their terms has not been paid over to Messiers Cyr and Barre. We play fair, and do as we say," continued Labadie, "and here is the money to cover our statement." Suiting the word to the deed, he slammed a roll of bills on the stage floor.

Attendants began to carry in the weights belonging to Cyr, which had remained parked in a wagon around the corner of the theatre. Mr. King looked questioningly at Cyclops and began to confer with him, but it was plain to see that the German was not going to have anything to do with Cyr or his weights. With emphatic headshaking and pounding of one fist into the palm of the other hand, he laid down the law to his manager and the theatrical manager and insisted that Cyr had no right upon the platform. The whole bunch argued and counter- argued, but nothing in the whole world could induce Cyclops to attempt a single lift with Cyr. Many a man with less self-control than Louis would have struck the German for the many scandalous things he had said about him, but Louis was ever a gentleman; nevertheless, the look of scorn that settled upon his face penetrated the case-hardened hide of Cyclops and seared his soul with shame. So tumultuous and threatening did the assemblage become towards the foreigners, that the theatrical management feared for the safety of the building as well as the person of the performers. Cyclops was obdurate; he would not lift, and as the fact was recognized, missiles began to float through the air and the curtain came down, leaving Louis the undisputed victor of the field.

It was an ignominious finish to the boastings of the trio who had acted without the least particle of sportsmanship. Knowing that Louis was absent, they deliberately took the unfairest advantage possible, hoping by such means to clean up and get away with the harvest of ill- gotten gains before Louis could return. But they played with a boomerang which came back at them and stripped them of any hope of popularity or success in America. They lived to regret their act, and although the two men, Cyclops and Sandowe, teamed together two or three years on the American stage, they were not successful. Cyclops returned to Europe little better off than when he came over. James Montgomery Irving settled down in New York, where he ran a gymnasium for many years. A year or two later, after the Montreal episode, Irving and Cyclops met Sebastian Miller and Otto Schmidt, winning a contest on their own tests, which consisted of lifts and tests of chain and stone-breaking. The victory is not one at which to marvel. If a man cannot beat his opponent on his own stuff, he cannot win on anything. Nothing could induce the pair to meet Miller and Schmidt on their set of tests. No, sir, they took no chances, although it is interesting to note that no one apart from Cyr lifted Cyclops' bell in America. Cyclops claimed that he lifted two hundred and eighty-six pounds two nights before this contest. Personally, I do not believe it, for the simple reason that Cyr said he later lifted the bell in private, when Cyclops was nightly claiming two hundred and eighty- six pounds for the lift and doubted if it weighed over two hundred and forty-five pounds. He ought to know; nevertheless, it was a lift that impressed the public and was the undoing of many a man who could trim Cyclops soundly on a general set of lifts. After the contest with Miller and Schmidt, nothing more was heard of them.

# CHAPTER IV

The sensational manner in which the big Montrealer unmasked the two rang around the world, and the Europeans and British began to marvel as to what kind of man Cyr was. Cyclops on his return to France told Professor Desbonnet that he never saw such a big man in all his life. He said that when Cyr confronted him on the night of October 28, 1891, the size of his arms and chest stupefied him. He further admitted that by the manner in which Cyr tossed around his weights he knew that Cyr had twice his strength, and he would only have made a bigger fool of himself than what he already had, if he had lifted against Cyr on the following night in Montreal, when Louis had all his weights carried on the stage. Desbonnet did not feel inclined to believe all that Cyclops told him of the St. Cyprien giant, for at that time Old France had a marvel of her own, a man of extraordinary proportions and over the average height — Apollon, the French giant. The Parisian professor was a little bit inclined to believe that Cyclops was offering an excuse for his defeat; but the splendid professor was to bow before the ponderous Louis in submission and recognition of a super force. Out of it all the mountain of strength received many pressing offers to perform in England. Louis was not quite ready to go, as he desired to fill more engagements in Canada and America before he took his leave for the land of the red and white rose. Greater than ever he felt the power of his conquest, and on every trial of force he strove to outrival his previous best performance. Big as he was, Louis was never lazy. He was a rare fighter. Put him up against something that was more difficult than he had encountered, and it was as though he was smitten upon the shoulder with the Titan rod. He would rise like a giant from his fastness and hurl himself against his material foe. There was no laying down for him. His eyes would snap with fire as his frame responded, and he has been known to lift until he bled from his exertions. His pupil, Horace Barre, whom he now included in his troupe, developed into a mighty man, and by many is believed to have been stronger than Cyr, but his blood was as water compared to that which flowed through the veins of Louis. He had not the sand in him to fight, and would quit before he would exert himself. Only on three or four occasions did he ever go his limit.

Actually he was lazier than the Parisian, Apollon; but not so with Louis. Tell him someone had done such and such a lift and Louis would immediately set himself to the task of scoring above it. Cyclops had spread the statement that his former partner, Sampson, could sustain the pull of two horses, one on either arm. Louis told his friends if such was the case, then he could hold the pull of four horses. On December 20, 1891, it was announced that the world's champion would do so at Sohmer Park, which was in those days the pleasure grounds of Montreal.

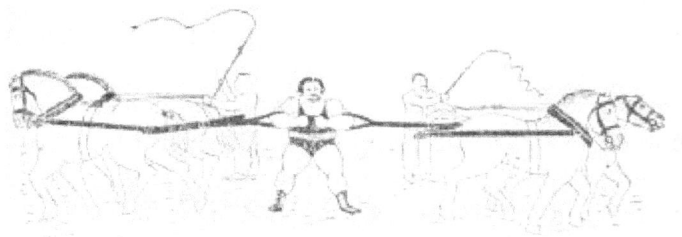

Before the eyes of 10,000 people, four huge draught horses were brought out fully harnessed with whiffletrees dragging on the ground. The horses were drawn off into pairs and Louis took up his stand between them. Around the fold of his huge upper arms was a heavy strap of leather, with a hook attached. To this hook the whiffletrees were hitched, while a groom stood at the head of each team. Louis then folded his great arms over his tremendous chest and spread his feet firmly apart. Satisfied as to his stance, he gave the signal to go and the grooms led the horses forward until they tightened in the traces. The grooms stepped aside and shouted to the horses to pull. With voice and cracking whips, they urged the powerful draught horses on. Nostrils distended and snorting they tugged forward, straining the muscles of their haunches so that they looked as though they would leap through the skin. Their well-shod feet dug deep into the ground as their backs flattened, but the resistance of one man held them until their hind feet slid back, piling up the earth. The cheering of the 10,000 watchers for Louis to hold 'em spurred the horses on with excitement to do their best; but their best was unavailing, as Louis stood like the rock of Gibraltar until the signal was given that he had won and the horses were released, trembling from their exertion.

After this wonderful feat he made ready his preparations for the overseas tour that was to take him to the then capital of the world.

He had long since decided that when he crossed the Atlantic Ocean he would be fortified by the knowledge within himself that his appearance and feats of manpower would be such as to administer a smashing blow to the foreign legions of iron men who had congregated on the little sea-girt isle of England. For no other reason had he delayed his departure from America. He desired time to study his act so that all the rough edges would be polished off, not so much for his own benefit as for that of his young protege, Horace Barre, who was much less of a finished performer. Many of the feats Louis and Barre were doing together were such that rhythm of movement and co-opera- tion of effort must be perfect. There must be no let-down there, for the big-hearted giant was fully aware how quickly the professional jealousy of the other strength artists would see and pick out any flaws. Then, he was fully alive to the scoffings of doubt that rumor had carried across the leagues of sea to him, circulated by the men who were each claiming to be stronger than the rest. Perhaps for the first time Louis began to analyze the actual possibilities of the strength that lay within him. Many, many hours he pondered over just how much he could do in this test or that, and as he arrived at various conclusions he worked like a horse to prove them. Every day he performed some startling feat, but never once did he reveal the fact. That was reserved for the time when he was to make his advent before his critics and the skeptics in London. That was to be the grand coupe, when his deeds alone would pronounce his superiority over all others, and be a fitting substantiation to back up the deposit he had placed with the "Sporting Life" for a contest with Sampson, the man who was formerly the senior partner in the Sampson-Cyclops act, when Sampson was hailed as the strongest human in the world. For Eugene Sandow, Louis had brought over his protege and team mate, Horace Barre, but neither was destined to meet either of those men. Such is fate. Man proposes, but God disposes. Still the months of assiduous toil were not to be in vain. They were to provide a greater triumph than the mere conquest of Sampson and Sandow would ever give. At the same time I know that Louis would have preferred to have met his adversaries in a physical contest, for if there was one thing genial Lou loved to do, it was to pit his powers against that of others.

December crept on and the waning days of 1891 began to close, opening a new gladness which seems to unfold with the coming of every new year. To the simple, superstitious souls of Cyre and Barre, the coming of the new year seemed like a good omen for them to embark upon their great adventure. They attended mass and the Christmas festivals, with the devotion common to the people who are born and reared in the land of churches, as Quebec is termed. Both men were devout Catholics and lived their lives treating others as they wished to be treated. It was upon this code that Louis built his ethics. He was the soul of honesty. Prior to his departure he told a close friend of his: "I am going over there to show the people what I can do. If any of those strong men feel that they are good enough to lift my weights, I want them to try, but I have no desire to talk about them or against them." How different is the philosophy of some men. He went to do and not to boast, and as you go with me through the scenes of his epoch-making British tour you will feel that he was qualified to repeat the memorable words of the great Caesar, who, fresh from his conquests, summed up everything in the three Latin words—"Veni, Vidi, Vici"— I came, I saw, I conquered.

On a snapping cold New Year's Day we find on the wharf at New York, two huge men with serious faces saying their "Au Revoirs" to all of their well-wishers. They were in the midst of a crowd of admirers until they stepped onto the ship that was to take them across the waters.

There are only a few months in the year which can be called pleasant to cross this briny stretch, and January was not one of them. Instead, any person will find the first two months of the year the very worst. All the fiendish elements of sea and sky seem to gather together during these months in one great orgy of devilish abandon, bent on the destruction of all things living. Barre did not need this point explained to him, for after the first day out at sea he became perfectly satisfied that it was so. For such a big, powerful man he was terribly afraid of the unseen, and every day of bad weather at sea impressed him as being so much worse than the day before. Although he was only a boy in his teens at this time, yet all through his life he was very superstitious. Dark places and night were filled with ghosts and rattling chains, so you can understand why he imagined that the chains of the devil were being wrapt around the boat at night, as the ship bulwarks creaked under the beating of wind and wave. Gladly would he have left the boat at any time and walked home if he could, but as the cliffs of old England were seen he began to feel better, and it was with a great sigh of relief that he stepped off the boat onto the dock at Liverpool. Do not think from this that Barre was cowardly. No, sir; not with anything he could see or knew was flesh and bone. He could fight like a bull dog. There are many people just like Barre, and I am purposely recounting this peculiarity in his moral make-up to show you that even strong men are human. It was in this characteristic that Cyr and Barre differed. Cyr was always an intrepid man. Positively fearless. To use a common expression, he feared nothing living or dead, and many were soon to know that Louis Cyr was not the backwoodsman from a country ridden with red savages that he had malignantly been reported to be.

His arrival was hailed with curiosity by the British people. The newspapers were filled with first impressions of the American strong man. So well written up were these impressions of the man and so vivid the interest aroused in a being who was described as being built like the side of a house, that everything bade fair for a mammoth attendance at his London debut. He was booked to appear at the Royal Aquarium, the largest place of amusement in England thirty-five years ago. It was within those same walls that all the famous men of might had been demonstrating their wares, breaking chains, bending iron and raising weights of great size. When weights were lacking platforms were brought forward, and horses and elephants used instead. This was the birthplace of the interest in the strong man that was rolling like a wave around the world and gaining extravagant recklessness at every turn. Within those same walls had been discharged volleys of challenges and counter-challenges— enough to shatter the place to atoms. The British mind was reeling with the question of Who Is Who, but the spell of the strong man was upon them, and their curiosity to see the long-haired giant from across the sea was tremendous. The opening night brought about a box-office jam. The phlegmatic Briton showed that when he was roused from his habitual manner of indifference he could display the same eagerness shown by the temperamental French Canadians, when they crashed the box office in their craze to see the Cyr-Cyclops clash in Montreal.

On the night of January 19th, 1892, five thousand people packed the Royal Aquarium in London, the largest .indoor crowd that had up to that time ever been in a theatre, and just as many were forced to remain outside. I believe that it was the most auspicious congregation of people to ever witness a strong act in the history of strongmanism. Statesmen, royalty, captains of commerce and great ecclesiastics that night rubbed shoulders on an equal basis with the factory workers and road sweepers of aristocratic England. The veneer produced by generations of civilizations fell away from them like a mantle of unreality. In all their spiritual nakedness they had gathered as man to man, to see THE MAN. The galaxy of strong men that crowded the boxes was greater than ever before or since to congregate before a brother strong man. If they only knew it, their numbered presence was a greater tribute to Cyr, and the belief in the little truthful voice sounding within them, that insisted THE MAN at last had come. There were the McCann brothers, fine, worthy strong men; Professor Szalay, the wonderful little dynamo of energy and enthusiasm, who was the hub of British strength activities; Monte Saldo, the Spencer brothers, Launceston Elliott, Charles Vanstittart, Sampson, and last, but not least, Professor Louis Attila with his famous protege, Eugene Sandow, among a hundred other iron tossers who waited with impatience through the other acts for the only one that could thrill them.

The curtain did not raise to the crescendo of voices that had greeted the towering form of Cyr throughout Canada and the United States. Instead there was an audible silence as the back curtain parted in the center, and the spotlight illuminated the giant frame that was posed in a natural attitude with feet apart, the right arm flexed across the chest and the left hand resting upon the left hip. All the audience could do was gaze and gasp. Even Sampson and Attila, who had both seen the giant form of Apollon, the Parisian, were stirred at the sight of this primitive looking creature. The tense silence was only broken as the manager of Cyr stepped forward and made his announcement, which in itself was another surprise. Free of any bombastic claims, he told his story simply. "Louis Cyr in America is accepted as the strongest man in the world, by rightly defeating all comers. Never has Cyr refused to meet any man, and we have come over to England on purpose to accept the challenges thrown out by all the strong men who are at the present time in this country. We have deposited one thousand pounds with the 'Sporting Life' to cover any amount that Sampson or Sandow wish to wager; Louis Cyr will meet any man at any time, preferably Sampson, who claims to be the strongest man in the world, or Eugene Sandow, who disputes Sampson's claims. We dispute the claims of any man to call himself the world's strongest man until he has met and defeated Louis Cyr. On the stage we have many weights which are open to the inspection of any man. I want any of you strong men to come up and test them. It is your privilege to weigh them, or try to lift them, so that you will know the poundages we name are right. Will any man care to test them?" This concluding shaft found no response, for not one among the gathering of strong men moved. Subconsciously they realized their inability to cope with the weights before them. Nevertheless, there were many among them who thought that Sampson or Sandow should have tried. At that time British opinions were divided as to the relative merits of Sampson and Sandow. The first named was by many preferred by reason of his great harness list performed the previous November, when he raised a total poundage of three thousand eight hundred and nine pounds on the same platform on which Louis now stood. Many favored Sandow by reason of his great bent press lift of two hundred and sixty-nine pounds. Neither man showed the least inclination to test the brawny Montrealer, not even when the crowd, released from its stupor, called on them to do so. Cyr accepted their reluctance as a silent challenge to prove himself, which was like a scourge to his spirit. With his ponderous stateliness he stepped forward and salaamed a courteous bow to the onlookers, and proceeded to unfold the fruits of his months of practice. Placed on his mettle, he plunged into his first lift with a vengeance. He meant to shock them all with a new record, and chose the one-arm lift for a start. The announcer cried out two hundred and fifty-eight pounds, and before the echo had reached the crowd that swarmed all over the gallery, Louis had made the lift with as much indifference as if it was naught. The big dumb bell was next made the equal of Sandow's record of two hundred and sixty-nine pounds, and as Louis stepped towards the lump of iron, a tensed expression was seen to settle upon the debonair countenance of Eugene. A heave and a toss, and the dumb bell was at the shoulder— silence followed so acute that the seconds in the theatre clock could be plainly counted as they ticked off. To the time of the ticking, the weight was steadily being raised. Not a falter. The big frame began to bend slightly sideways, but the legs remained firm and straight as the weight passed the crown of the head. Never for an instant did any one strong man shift his gaze. Fascinated, dumfounded, each leaned forward following the weight in its journey. From excitement Professor Szalay rose to his feet as though drawn by the impelling influence of mesmerists hands, while Sandow gripped the sides of the chair he sat in until his knuckles gleamed whitely through the skin, as he saw the final stage of the lift that equaled his own world's record. The throng rose, exploding into tumultuous cheers in genuine appreciation of a magnificent deed. But they were to see more yet. The bell was loaded a third time, and rolled forward as the announcer roared in a stentorian voice "Two hundred and seventy-three and one-quarter pounds." Sandow settled himself back into his seat. More quickly than any other had he detected the unrevealed powers of Cyr as he had watched the second lift made. He had foresight, and he knew that his own record mark, bar accidents, was doomed. Others began to think Louis was biting off a little too much, and then there were the enthusiasts who were so lost in admiration that they were willing to believe that he had no limitations. The newspaper clippings that I have of that time claim that Cyr pulled the final weight up to the shoulder in one clean movement and then pressed it overhead. He certainly pressed it, and performed the lift in the same manner that he had done the last. To those who are not so familiar with strong-man stunts, they may think that four and one-quarter pounds difference does not mean much, but there is a world of difference in the way the two men lifted. When Sandow made his great lift, England marveled, but Europe shrugged her shoulders and said that was not a genuine lift. I am not going to argue about whether it is a genuine lift or not, for anything that requires handling calls for strength. The screw lift, as the bent press was called in those days, was new to them, but the science involved in the lift that enabled a smaller man to catch up to a big man did not allow most big men to employ it. To stand and just shove a weight overhead requires about fifty to seventy-five per cent more strength according to the amount lifted. It was in this latter manner that Cyr put up the frightful weight of two hundred and seventy-three and one-quarter pounds. It was impossible for him to do the lift like Sandow, who had improved upon the style used by the first demonstrators, Pennell and Attila. Cyr was too huge a man for that. For that reason the Europeans could better appreciate the enormity of the lift. By this I do not mean to say that the English would not appreciate Cyr's great lift. They could, and they did. That one lift crowned him Lord of All that night and they were with him to a man. The professional strong man began to realize there was more truth than poetry in the way the giant Canadian had polished off Cyclops. No raillery left their lips about the bulk of the man before them. The size of Cyr's legs was too convincing. They were interested in what was to happen next. Next was a two-hands lift to the shoulder in one movement and press slowly overhead a bar bell of three hundred and one pounds. There was not a man there who could even jerk the weight overhead, a movement that carries the weight to arms' length a third easier, and to pull it in to the shoulders with one movement was infinitely much more difficult for any of them. The first stage of the lift was a huge surprise to them, for they could not believe a man of such a body weight could lean over far enough to perform the initial movement. Cyr realized that he had them all stumped, and went on to show them he could toss weights around in faster movements than just press lifts. A large, ugly, solid dumb bell of one hundred and seventy- four pounds was swept off the floor to right arm's length with no ceremony at all, to be instantly repeated with the left hand. The arm was kept straight at right angles to the body all the time in a perfect swing lift, as we now term it. The only difference was that he did not bend the legs at any time as he swept the weight from the floor overhead. The next feat was a greater surprise. He took a weight of one hundred and four and one-half pounds and held it out with one hand so that it lay level with the shoulder in a crucifix lift. To show his absolute control over the weight at this awkward angle, he held it there a few moments and then brought it back to the shoulder in the same parallel line that he had thrust the weight out in. From this feat he passed on to one that he had often performed before, shouldering the barrel of cement that weighed three hundred and fourteen pounds without using the aid of his knees. Then he walked off the stage with it as though it was empty, and returned to dazzle the audience with a stupendous one-finger lift off the floor with five hundred and fifty-one pounds. An unbelievable feat to the audience, but they rapidly became convinced when they saw none of the watching strong men make any effort to deny it one way or the other.

There was a greater reason for Louis' method of performance on this night than you can see by just reading the order of the feats. The strong men saw that the routine Cyr had mapped out took in all the feats of strength which separately were their individual boasts and specialties. Therefore each lift made by Cyr tumbled down a castle upon each one of them. It required no mind reader among them to figure out that if Cyr could beat one record after another in one nightly performance, he could positively do much better if he specialized upon each lift separately.

The next feat of Cyr was his last, and, to use a twentieth-century term, it was a greater knockout than the lift he opened his show with. He called for any number of men to come upon the stage, and from them he selected the biggest, and placed them all upon a heavy platform that was resting upon two trestles. Louis then crept under the platform and placed his back under the center of the board, and before the astounded eyes of everyone he raised the load clear off the trestles and held it thus supported upon the broad of his back with no other aid but that of his mighty body. The total weight was estimated at three thousand six hundred and thirty-five pounds. This was the one feat that thrilled England and the one by which he is remembered.

The curtain went down that night in a perfect triumph for the visitor. Every other man was forgotten. All that could be heard was Cyr, Cyr, Cyr. None of the men of might accepted Louis' defy, nor did they throw any challenge in the direction of the overwhelming presence. Like Cyclops, Miller and Sandowe, Sampson and Eugene Sandow were awed into silence. Never had they seen such a sized man. The depth of his chest, the span of his back and those legs and arms. "My God," they cried— "He is tremendous"—that is what they all said. Verbally, they both claimed to be the world's strongest man on the strength of their one pet lift, but in their hearts they knew there were many other men much stronger than they. In Germany, Hans Beck was nationally acclaimed the strongest Teuton, and Europe accepted August Johnson as the strongest of Europeans.

France was acclaiming the colossal Apollon, and in Britain, Donald Dinnie was considered a fitting opponent for any man. As a matter of fact, Louis Attila was a stronger all-around man than his pupil, Eugene Sandow.

# CHAPTER V

But Cyr proved in one night that he could outlift them all. The only dark horse was August Johnson, a man who was very quiet. In actual contests, and by his feats, he was more entitled to call himself the champion of the world than Sampson or Sandow, but he never did. His modesty was superior to that. He actually was the only man to place down a wager with the honest intention of lifting against the great Canadian, and their contest which later took place in Chicago was the greatest in history, as I will relate in its proper place.

Dinnie was an exceedingly strong man and carved a career for himself that has never been equaled for all-round ability. He was one of those Scotchmen who are proud of the heather, and he had a great opinion of himself. He believed that no man was as good as a Scotchman, and he was the king of Scotch strong men. In his swinging kilt he was truly a magnificent sight. The type of a Scotchman you read about but rarely ever see. I remember meeting him when he was well up in his seventies, and he was then a fine specimen of manhood, hale, and hearty. In those days he was living his glorious youth, just as Cyr was, and in throwing the hammer, putting the shot, jumping, tossing the caber, he had them all stopped. Apart from this, he was a superb wrestler and had outlifted most of the strong men that ever dared pit their strength against him. He was very powerful in lifting weights off the ground, and also in "muscling out," feats which you will recognize that Cyr was most capable of doing.

Proof of his great man power is evidenced by his ability to carry a huge stone with a ring in it that some of the world's strongest men could scarcely move off the ground. How much it weighed, I am sorry to say I do not know. Somehow this cynical Scot found himself drawn to the great Canadian, and the formal meeting between Kelt and

Gaul was a study in character. Dinnie invited Cyr to his home, and he afterwards admitted that Cyr was the only man that ever impressed him at first sight Immediately the canny Scot showed Louis the great stone, and characteristically exclaimed, "I gae nae mon credit wi' being stronger than I, 'less he can do what I can't." Substantiating his words, he raised the stone and walked with it. Louis did not wait for any invitation, but, fully dressed, he raised the stone and carried it like a sack of salt. Dinnie exclaimed aloud as he saw the ease with which Cyr walked away three times the distance he had gone with the stone. "Mon, mon, ye should hae bane a Scot," to which Louis naively replied with a slight bow, "M'sier, I am thankful to be a French Canadian." A great friendship grew up between these two men of opposite natures that never wavered throughout their lives. Dinnie always said that Cyr had the greatest bodily strength of any man he had ever seen. Donald had toured around the world and had seen 'em all; besides, had he not taken part in over a thousand contests! By reason of his own great conquests, he was more fitting to judge than any other man in Britain.

Feted by Britain's "first gentleman" and peer of Sportsmen, the Prince of Wales, who later became King Edward VII, the visitor from New France stepped from one glory to another. His mild demeanor and kindly smile won him friends wherever he went, and every day he found the capital of the world a more entrancing place. Its great cathedrals and history of men of great French lineage breathed something of his forefathers.

Born of a simple faith, he was one of those rare individuals who could give any one the full benefit of a doubt, and being a truthful man, he never expected others to doubt his word. Consequently, he was shocked on being adjudged otherwise at one of his London performances. He had gone through his regular routine and come to his great dumbbell lift, in which he pushed overhead with one hand two hundred and fifty pounds at every performance.

The announcer gave out the poundage and Louis pushed, but somehow it seemed to go up far too quickly for some of the gallery gods, who shouted out, "Garn, Mister, tain't no sich weight." Louis was shocked into stillness while the weight was hardly past half way up, and he stared into the audience with surprise stamped all over his face. The fact that he now held the weight so indifferently seemed to make the lift more unbelievable, so that the chorus more mockingly repeated themselves. Speechless for the moment, Louis lowered the weight to his side and blankly stared up at his inquisitors. Then it dawned on him that these people were trying to make him out a faker. As he found his voice, he indignantly roared out his defiance, "Who are you to say that this weight is not what I say, when you have not the courage to come down and try to lift it. I will give you one hundred pounds if you can come down and lift it as I do. Please come down, as I do not want you to doubt my feat. The money is waiting for you." Thoroughly incapable of backing their words, they shut up, but all this time Louis had been standing with the dumbbell hanging at arms' length by his side; and without bending his body he gave the bell a slight arm swing that took it to the shoulder from the hanging position, and from there he pressed it overhead for the second time that night. Charles Vanstittart, the man who was known as the man with the iron hand, when recounting this incident, said that it was the greatest feat of strength he ever witnessed. Well; just imagine how great was his arm strength to slowly lower the weight and hold it by his side while keeping up a flow of talk, and then practically curl it and press it overhead for the second time, all inside of a couple of minutes. If Vanstittart had not been the one to tell it, I doubt whether I would have cared to believe it.

I have spoken so much of Louis' great strength that now I must tell you of his great weakness—eating. His excuse for eating so much was that his.great expenditure of strength required it. That was just his joke, though, for he was a slave to the table all his life. He could eat more than four ordinary men at one sitting, and took a keen delight watching the amazement creep over the waiter's face when he turned in his order at the hotel. Six pounds of meat at one meal was nothing for him. He could devour that for breakfast. Next to a lifting contest, he loved an eating contest best, and any man who thought he could tuck more food under his belt than Louis was an agreeable friend with an agreeable pastime, and the question must be settled by a bet and a trial. Many a gourmand has gone away wiser in head and lighter in pocket after a meat-and-potato contest with the giant Louis. His homecomings were always a feast, with everything done up royally on the table.

Although Louis had turned out to be a nomad like Hercules of old, yet he loved the land of his nativity, and in days of rest turned to his beautiful farm that was situated outside of Montreal. On it were only the best cattle, and among these was a beautiful gray horse with all characteristics of a thoroughbred. This big driving gray horse was his pride, and was a gift to him from the Marquis of Queensbury. The latter was a peer who had sprung from a long line of sportsmen, and the Marquis about whom I am speaking was a worthy son of a great father. While Louis was in England, the Marquis made the request for Cyr to perform in private before him and a number of other notable British sportsmen. Gentleman Louis had not the heart to refuse, after being treated so magnificently by them all, and had all of his paraphernalia sent out so he could put on his entire show. Louis was magnificently received, and went through all of his stuff with gusto. He always did his best when he knew he had an appreciative audience. They marveled at his strength, and two very prominent medical men were astounded to find his flesh to be so steel-like to their touch. As they were about to adjourn to the sumptuous repast the Marquis had prepared for Louis as the guest of honor, Louis said, "But, Marquis, I need just a little more exercise to get up an appetite. If you have a pair of horses that can pull, I will give them a chance to test my strength." Immediately they all adjourned to the stable, and the Marquis had the grooms lead out a handsome pair of driving grays that weighed about twenty-three hundred pounds. He smiled as he said to Louis, "If you succeed in holding those horses to a standstill with one hitched on either arm and each pulling in opposite directions, I will make you a present of your choice." The guests became greatly excited as they saw the huge Goliath stand between the horses, and many tried to persuade him to desist from a feat that appeared dangerously foolhardy to them, but Louis was in the throes of a physical combat which was the fire of his fibre. He threw back his head and laughed aloud in wild abandon as he felt the passion of combat surging through his blood. He gave the word, and the grays bounded away together, snorting with the discharge of all their thoroughbred power; but Louis held them as powerless as Prometheus chained to the rock. For all their herculean efforts, a mightier being held them. Louis said afterward that it was the hardest pull he had ever sustained. The Marquis and his friends were thrilled with delight, and joyfully the British peer asked Louis to make his choice before the trembling beasts were led away. After they had partaken of their repast and prepared to leave, one of Louis' attendants led away with them the gray thoroughbred, which could be seen for many years after on Louis' farm in Canada, where it always had an affectionate, loving master.

The enormity of Louis' lifts impressed the public mind; yet the average theatregoer saw no beauty in his colossal build. The type of physique exemplified by Eugene Sandow naturally appealed to them more. Yet who will deny that the delicate beauty of the poplar is not lost in the terrific grandeur of the mighty oak. Who would dare to compare the lovely Hudson with the roar and the roll of the giant Mississippi. You may gaze down the valleys of New Hampshi re, but the majestic glory of the Grand Canyon is what will awe you with its enormity. People found in Cyr much of the primeval ruggedness which the great Northwest country breeds, and that generations of conventionality had stripped them of.

His mighty frame with its immense back suggested Atlas as he must have been when he held the world upon his shoulders. Only Hercules could relieve Atlas of his load, but this earthly Atlas of the nineteenth century looked in vain for an Hercules to compare with. Sampson and his minions faded into obscurity, and the light of Sandow visibly paled. Not until the Gaulish lord of Ironia bade farewell to England and Europe did Eugene regain his popularity.

Queen Victoria received her colonial subject and showered gifts upon him until it was said that no man received such honors as the giant, Louis Cyr.

France; old France; the land of his ancestors was his next destination. Gay Paris looked askance at the man whose forefathers had shaken off the dust of France from their shoes for a newer country generations ago. Then they had one among them who was hailed as the greatest of French strong men, and, with the typical French mind, they dubbed others as imposters in their claim to the world's strong-man title. Professor Desbonnet was one who believed the millennium of strong men had arrived with Apollon, in whom it was invested; and he did not for one moment believe the statements of Cyclops and others concerning Cyr. Even the reports from England had only made him smile, and said, "How can they judge of the strong man when they have never seen one." Truly he was justified in some of his beliefs, for those who had come before Cyr in Britain were as pygmies compared to Luis Uni. But when Cyr stepped before Desbonnet stripped for action, the great professor was more appalled than any other man. So egotistical was he in his belief that anything bigger than Apollon was impossible. Desbonnet fell back as though he had been struck a blow; he reeled under the im mensity of the man before him, and could only whisper, "Mon Dieu! What a man." The titanic proportions of Apollon fell away as he saw those mighty limbs that sprung from the trunk of a giant oak. Desbonnet in his book, "Le Rois de Force" (The Kings of Strength) names Cyr and Apollon the super-men of the ages, and says that he never saw or could believe it possible for a man to grow legs of such girth, and a chest so massive that it looked like a cliff surmounting the sea. The arms, the back, the everything. Yes; and they had the steel within them. Cyr brought the people of France to his feet and proved to them that of all strong men he was the strongest. Satisfied with his con- quests, he turned his face homeward, leaving a host of friends and good fellowship behind him that has been handed down from father to son. Some years ago when I was among them, I chanced to hear some men talk of the great strong men they had met, when one man rose and said loudly, "I met the greatest of them all and shook his hands. I knew the great Louis Cyr." No one denied the man. Despite their pride in meeting others, they felt that by not seeing Cyr they had lost much.

# CHAPTER VI

We next find Cyr back in America, drawing the eyes of the world to his great back-lifting feat, on May 27th, 1895, at the museum of Austin and Stones in Boston, Mass. Previously he had made the statement that on this night he was going to outlift any back-lift record he had ever made, and the weight would not be under four thousand pounds. The place was so crowded that many people were turned away unable to get any further than the entrance.

The hour arrived, and the indomitable Cyr ascended the stairs leading to the exhibition platform with a firm step, his heart light, and his general demeanor that of a man imbued with the idea that he was about to perform the most remarkable feat of his life. He paused as the cheering ceased and cast a cursory glance over the audience. His eyes fell upon one giant form here, and another there, and still another, until eighteen bulky men were called out and stood beside the champion. Most men would have weakened at the task before them, but the Canadian wore the same self-satisfied smile as he motioned the men to take up their appointed place upon the lifting platform. I remember a Boston press report of that night, stating that as Cyr got beneath the load everything became so tensed in silence that the munching of a diminutive monkey up in one corner of the hall could be plainly heard—it is strange how these incidental things will impress themselves upon your mind on such memorable occasions, but they do, very vividly.

Louis prepared himself for the grand effort. With feet firmly spaced and hands gripping the oaken bench in front of him, he began to lift. There was a creak, a strain, but the platform did not budge. He moved his back a little, and the spectators, drawn by the movement, unconsciously moved with him. Louis wore a determined look and started again. His frame quivered and the muscles on his arms and legs seemed to draw the skin taut as they leaped to the task. Would he succeed? Anxious inquiry was depicted upon many faces. The platform creaked like a rusty hinge. It began to move. Again it moved. Up it was going, sure enough. A mighty shout tore from the throats of every watcher as they saw the terrific load of four thousand three hundred pounds suspended in mid-air, supported upon the back of the invincible Cyr. The crowd continued to pour out its compliments as Cyr, flushed more with the recognition of his admirers than the exertion, stepped out from beneath the load. This was the greatest back lift ever recorded, and the best he ever did. It was a record not forgotten, and as a token of recognition the sportsmen of Boston made him a beautiful presentation before he left the city.

Cyr also received the Richard K. Fox, Police Gazette Belt, which pronounced the great French Canadian as the undisputed champion of the world. The years of 1892 and 1896 were the two red-letter years of his great career. The latter years we are now in and find the genuine Sandow over in America making the claim in a New York paper that he was the strongest man in the world. Louis happened to be in Philadelphia when he heard this. He immediately set out for New York and walked into the editorial offices of the paper that had published the Sandow statement, and slammed down $500.00 as a deposit to cover any amount and publicly accepted the challenge. By the side of his wager he laid his Police Gazette Belt Trophy and said, "Let Sandow take this from me if he is man enough." The truth was Louis was sore at the small man's assumption. Needless to say, Sandow declined, and America never took Sandow seriously as a real strong man while they did bow to his beautiful physique and superb showmanship. Barre had left Cyr, and the latter filled his place with an all Cyr act. He had a brother who was thirteen years younger than himself named Peter, who at the time was just nineteen.

There was a world of difference in the build of the two. Peter was very tall and only weighed 154 pounds, but he was remarkably strong, and was unbeatable at his weight in straddling barrels of sand and water, and lifting them off the floor. Peter could clean and jerk with two hands two hundred and fifty-one pounds, and made a one-arm lift of one hundred and ninety-six pounds with a dumb bell. In conjunction with this act Louis had his nine-year-old daughter, a sweet-faced, charming little girl who was a real chip off the old block. This little Amazon used to go through a few stunts with her father, and you can imagine how popular she was.

Talk about the law of opposites, but Louis' marriage was it. Just as Louis was big, so was his wife little. Never did this worthy madam weigh over one hundred pounds, but she ruled the heart of the great-souled iron man. Madame Cyr never wearied of watching him perform, and became the inspiration of some of his greatest feats. She was with him on the memorable night of March 31, 1896 when he made his great two-arm clean and jerk record of three hundred and forty-seven pounds, a world's record. The newspapers of that time said that Louis swept the weight off the floor with a rush, and with hardly a perceptible stop at the shoulders took it to arms' length. Whether he did it or not, I know Louis knew no science. There was no dipping or squatting under his lifts. Just a heave, and the rest was finished with a push out.

The next day, April the first, the unforgetable conflict between the giant of America and the extraordinary August Johnson, of Sweden, hailed as the strongest man in Europe! Oh boy; don't you get a great kick out of the proximity of events. Imagine the night before he meets the Lion of Scandinavia. He does his best in an exhibition and staggers the inhabitants of the world of weights with his record two-arm jerk overhead of three hundred and forty-seven pounds. What was the morrow to him! Oh, well, the day would take care of itself surely. So would he. He was always filled with confidence; but when you consider how other men rest and nurse themselves prior to a contest, you cannot help but admire this bear of a man.

Chicago was the scene of his last great feat, and was the scene of his clash with Johnson. Never was he any fitter than the night of April first, weighing in at two hundred and seventy pounds stripped, the lightest body weight of his career. So finely trained was he, that for the first time people beheld the massive boney scaffold of his huge frame and marvelled. Some tell me that his wrist measured a little over twelve inches, although it looked twice the size of mine, which is eight inches and a half. In Johnson, Cyr met the foeman most worthy of his steel, and a man who by reason of the great courage he showed in their contest endeared himself to the heart of the Canadian. Louis always claimed that Johnson was the strongest man he ever met in contest. The Swede was a large, finely built man of over two hundred pounds, with a pair of twenty-eight inch thighs and the rest of his measurements in proportion. He was the first man in the world ever to do a two hands clean and jerk with three hundred and twenty-eight pounds, and later raised three hundred and thirty pounds in the same manner. On October 16, 1892, in St. Petersburg, Russia, he made a one-arm press of two hundred and fifty-five pounds, using a dumb bell. He was at various times associated with Waklund and Hjalmar Lundin, two Swedes, who were possessed of enormous natural strength. Johnson was unusual in his day for strong men; he was reticent and mild natured, more like Cyr. Despite the fact that he had met the best men in Europe in open contests, he never once styled himself other than "Champion weight lifter of the world." He even dropped this title when he lost to Cyr.

Johnson and Cyr met for a side wager of $1000.00 each, to be contested on a series of lifts that consisted of bar-bell and dumb-bell lifting, with one and two hands, in both press and jerk lifts, muscling out weights, and also swinging a dumb bell off the floor to arms' length. These, with some one and two-hand dead lifting off the floor, without the use of harness, made up the entire program. They battled away until one o'clock in the following morning when Johnson, beaten on every lift, quit. He had fought so hard that his hands and fingers were blistered and raw, but Louis was no better off, for his fingers were split and bled freely from the strenuous task. His antagonist had run him so tight on most lifts, that the battling demon within him was aroused as never before. The Canadian was leading by two hundred pounds when the Swede quit exhausted, knowing it was hopeless to continue; but the lust of the battle was upon Louis, who fighting from every fibre of his perspiring body would not quit.

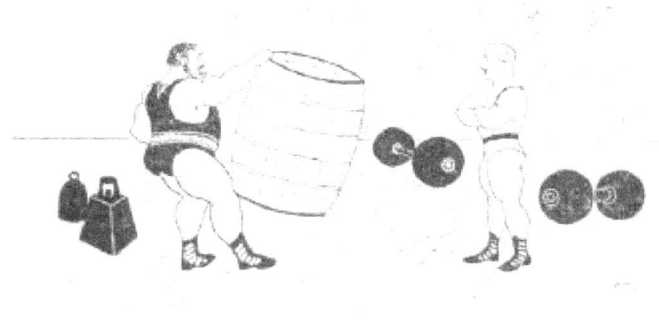

The most notable of his lifts was a repetition of his great two hands jerk of three hundred and forty-seven pounds. Johnson made a one- hand dead lift with a dumb bell of four hundred and seventy-five pounds, using an inch and a half bar. On the same bar Louis raised five hundred and twenty-five pounds. Although Johnson's withdrawal gave the victory to Cyr, yet the Montrealer decided that once and for all he was going to show the world that he alone was the supreme lord of strong men. From the night of April first until May eighth he conducted a strength fest all of his own, during which time he made some wonderful lifts, besides duplicating all of his previous records. The best of his feats were performed on the nights of May seventh and eighth as follows: a crucifix lift, using ninety-seven and one-quarter pound dumb bell in the right hand and eighty- eight pounds in the left hand. He pushed to arms' length a dumb bell of one hundred and sixty-two and one-half pounds with one hand thirty-six times in succession, a feat which proves he could have easily surpassed the world's one-arm military press record of one hundred and fifty-eight pounds by Barre if he had wanted. With either hand he made a dumb bell swing with one hundred and eighty-eight and one-half pounds, and a one-hand dumb bell clean and press with straight legs of two hundred and fifty-eight pounds. He made a one-finger lift of five hundred and fifty-two and one-half pounds, which was to be eclipsed on the following night, as also was his one-hand lift of nine hundred and eighty-seven pounds, done without any artificial help, or with the help of his knees. This was followed by what the newspaper reports call a two hands dead lift of one thousand eight hundred and ninety- seven and one-quarter pounds, but we would term it a hand-and-thigh lift. Next he shouldered a barrel filled with sand and water that weighed four hundred and thirty-three pounds, using the right hand without the help of the knees. Then it is claimed that he muscled-out with the right hand a dumb bell of one hundred and thirty-one and one-quarter pounds and held it there for five seconds before he brought it back to the shoulder. The next night (May eighth) a great gathering of prominent Chicago business men attended, the Reverend Father Boudreau, of Long Island, acting as chairman. They verify the following lifts: one-hand dead lift, with no other aid, of nine hundred and eighty-eight pounds—a duplication of his crucifix lift of the night before, and repetition lifting with the one hundred and sixty-five pound dumb bell. This night he shouldered, with the right arm, a barrel of iron and gravel weighing four hundred and forty-five pounds, taking hold only by the chines of the barrel. He imitated his one-hundred and thirty-one and one-quarter pound one-hand muscle-out and finished up with a one-finger lift of five hundred and fifty-eight pounds.

These feats were his great wind-up and the crowning features of his tourney of strength that had commenced as a lad of sixteen. Only on one more instance have we any record of him doing anything better; when appearing at Austin-Stones, in Boston, the next year he jerked from the shoulder three hundred and fifty pounds.

No man ever has accomplished such wonderful lifting over so many consecutive lifts as Cyr did night after night. No wonder Johnson said, "I can out-lift any man in the world, but it is impossible for any man to outlift that elephant."

No other conquests were in sight, so literally smothered in glory Louis laid back upon his well earned laurels. He began to team again with Horace Barre, for Barnum and Bailey's Circus. One of their most impressive feats was a back lift. One man got under each end of the platform and raised together thirty people. Their act was wound up in a very spectacular way. A platform was carried into the center of the sawdust ring with a number of chairs placed side by side along the full length of the platform. At each end was a pair of hand grips, behind which one of them stood facing its entire length, and the other backed up to his end. As the circus band struck up the grand march, each man took hold with his hands, and together lifted the entire weight free of the ground, and out of the circus arena they marched with their load.

Barre did not stay in the show business very steadily, nor very long. Despite his great natural strength he was not a success. There are some who say that Horace was a stronger man than Cyr, but he never proved it. No doubt he did some remarkable lifting; yet there was nothing about his lifts that Louis could not do. Often when they were training together, Louis would outlift Horace over a set of lifts so badly that Horace would quit. He lacked the fire that would make him a great fighter in any tough corner. Louis asked for nothing better than a tight struggle. The harder it was the better he liked it, and the more he lifted. Not for a moment do I wish to detract from the strength of Barre, for I believe he stood next to Cyr as the most formidable strong man of his day; but when all is said and done, Cyr was the strongest of the two, taking one lift with another. If Barre had had the same enthusiasm as Cyr for physical contest, some wonderful results would have been recorded. I believe feats of strength would have been registered on many tests that would have stood forever. However, it is fate that juggles with us, and not us with it. If fate did not play a hand in the game of life, things would be horribly stereotyped.

Louis had made a fortune, and he began to drift away from regular theatrical performance, spending his time with a few exceptions between his saloon and farm. Perhaps if Louis had stayed in the business, more would have been heard of Barre; unfortunately, Barre was easy prey for unscrupulous business men. When he gave up "the road," as show people say, he accepted a post as warden in a Montreal prison, but he and Louis remained bosom pals throughout their lives and often lived their adventures together over many a groaning board of food. In eating, as in lifting Barre was a close second to Louis. I heard that one time they had an eating match to be decided by which could devour a twenty-two pound suckling pig the quickest, and they say that Louis was done when Horace was little more than half way through. That this should have been their weakness is to be deplored, as it was the means of their death. While Louis was showing, he mastered this weakness, or I might better say his love to display his strength was stronger than his weakness. After he dropped away from active training he let himself go; yet you must never lose sight of the fact that strength must have an outlet. He had led a very strenuous life, using his strength for a living as others use their hands, and others their head. His new life was too inactive for his immense reserve of manpower, which had to be taken care of somehow. The unfortunate thing, as I see it, is that he should have allowed his natural failing for eating to provide the substitute for exercise. I am not blaming him. Why should I? We all have some weakness to which we submit, and because the other fellow's fault is not ours is no reason why we should condemn him. It is a natural weakness for us all to see the faults in others quicker than in ourself. All I have to say is if the majority of people were as clean living as the big souled Canadian, the world would be much better to live in. He alone paid the price, no one else suffered.

In the days of Cyr's activities, it was customary for strength athletes to offer a certain amount of money to any man who could duplicate their lifts. Often the money had been won by some local athlete, but rarely had it been paid. Louis carried a monetary challenge with his act, offering $100.00 to any man who could do any one lift in his performance, and $1000.00 to the one who could follow him throughout the whole routine. Naturally you will say he was safe enough, but there was one time that he had to lose $100.00 to a man named Therrien, of Michigan, who succeeded in duplicating one of his stunts. Which particular stunt it was, I do not recall, but I know he was the only one who ever was successful, and he was the only man I ever knew who received his money. Without any quibble Louis ordered his manager to pay Therrien the sum of $100.00 right there and then, while he shook hands with the man from Michigan. Four-square to all the winds, Louis sought no loop holes to four-flush the man out of what he was entitled to. However, many would-be Samsons got badly fooled, and it really was funny to see how eager every locality was to drag out its hero to match this sturdy son of Anak. Cyr was the first that I ever remember to leave any of his weights outside the place where he performed. He had a great big dumb bell that weighed around two hundred and fifty pounds, and the handle on it was monstrously large. Thousands of huskies tried it, but all they had to show for their vain attempts were bursted coat seams and broken belts. Clothes were worn tighter-fitting then than now, and any time of the day you cared to visit the scene of the giant dumb bell, you could see buttons fly, or find plenty scattered around on the ground, the sequel to the many vain attempts. But Louis was cute, and just to make his act a little more spicy, he would stick around until the last minute when everybody had tried, then walk through the throng up to the bell and pick it up with one hand as though it was a satchel, and walk up the steps, into the theatre and all the way back stage with no further ado beyond leaving the crowd gaping. Louis said he never saw any man lift it off the ground single-handed.

You can readily see that the strong-man profession has a humorous side to it as well as its serious encounters. It was when he was in Chicago that he was mistaken for a fat man by the doorkeeper of the theatre. This latter person happened to be rather young, and at an age when he believed nobody could put anything over on him. So it was with a scornful eye that he looked over the massive bulk of humanity that stood before him asking admittance to see the manager of the theatre. "Would you kindly tell M'sier that it is Louis Cyr?" he asked of the doorman. "You, Louis Cyr! Yeh; Fatty. So'm I," he grinned, stuffing his hands deep into the pockets of his pants as he lay back lazily against the wall. Louis quickly appraised the young fellow and smiled as he further insisted, but the other was obdurate. "You may be fat enough," he continued, "but you ain't big enough to be Louis Cyr. Now go away and play, the police force is too busy to turn out and cart an elephant like you to the hospital." Louis decided he had done all the talking he was going to, and started for the door that led to the manager's room. "Say, Tubby, you can't go in there," the doorkeeper yelled as he interposed himself between Louis and the door. Calmly the big man thrust out his giant hand and grabbed the young man by the clothes, lifting him clear off the ground. The doorman went pop-eyed and speechless, as Louis marched along with him tucked under his arm without any effort, finally depositing him with a sudden drop on the floor, as he stepped through the door into the manager's room.

A friend of mine told me that he and Louis were walking through the streets of Boston, when they came across a great commotion made by two teamsters who were trying their best to unlock the hind wheels of their wagons, which had become locked together. In spite of all their swearing, lashing the horses and their "Gee hawing," they got no further out of their trouble. My friend said that Louis placed his back under the tail end of one wagon and lifted it clear of its tangle, then with a step and a toss he heaved the wagon sideways, thus unlocking the locked situation. Done so quickly it took the people's breath, and they dispersed laughing, as people generally do when they see something done by one when the efforts of many had been resisted.

Oscar Matthes, the great little wizard of strengthdom, was a wonderful pal of Louis, and whenever the latter went to Boston they were together as much as possible. The affinity of extremes again appealing to the heart. Oscar was a foot shorter than Louis, and over 200 pounds lighter. They must have attracted some attention, all right, but so wrapped up were they in each other that little they cared at what amused others. Oscar told me that he saw Louis make a perfect two-hands military press with three hundred pounds, and that his three hundred and forty-seven pound two-arm clean and jerk record was a straight-legged press. He claimed that Louis could not jerk. I do know that Louis certainly never tried to jerk a weight the way lifters of today do. All he seemed to me to do to get a start was to shake his body like a huge St. Bernard dog, and the rest was truly finished with a press out of the arms. I have seen Louis place a fifty-pound block weight on the palm of his hand, with the arm bent at the elbow in the position a man is when half way through on an arm curl to the shoulder. On the top of the first he placed another, and then another until he had four balanced, then he would walk around the room and replace them on the floor as gently as though they were eggs. Such an arm! I can see it yet. Shades of Hercules! I cannot explain it.

# CHAPTER VII

I never will forget the first time I met him. It was very incidental and came at an age when first impressions are etched with vivid distinction upon the mind. You never forget. I had been standing at the corner of one of the cross streets of Notre Dame, about a block away from Place D'Armes, for about fifteen minutes, waiting for a pal who showed no signs of turning up. In fact, he had told me not to wait any later than eight o'clock, and it was then ten minutes after. Why I stood there so long I do not know. The night was cold, and the street so ill lit that it was almost in complete darkness. I guess I was in one of those retrospective moods of mine with nothing to do and all night to do it in. When I arrived I had noticed across the way what looked to be the end of a lighted cigar stuck in someone's mouth. The person was so hidden by the greater darkness of the doorway in which he stood that I could not see who it was, or what it was. In consequence, the lighted cigar appeared glaringly visible. I would watch it gleam and dull as the smoker puffed and relaxed on it, and all the time my interest grew. I can remember as though it was today, how I stood trying to pierce the darkness with a curiosity that made me think of what Ella Wheeler Wilcox said about the fascination in all human beings to raise the veil to peer into the unseen. Perhaps this reads queerly to you, as you may wonder what on earth is there to the lighted end of a cigar. Not much, as a rule, I'll admit, but there was this time. The light vanished and I still lingered. Presently a voice spoke—"Bon Soir, M'sier. Quelle heure est-il?" (which apart from bidding you a good night means he wants to know the time). I told him; then he asked me for a light, and I had to apologize for not having one. When I told the stranger I did not smoke he asked me with a friendly laugh if I were an athlete. Well, you can figure what happened after that. One thing led to another, which climaxed with his asking me if I knew personally the great Louis Cyr, with whom he was well acquainted. Up until then I had never seen Cyr, as I was quite young, and being a real enthusiast in body culture had never dreamed of frequenting saloons. Anyhow, the upshot was we started for Louis' place with me all a,thrill. Happily, it was too early for the regular nightly gathering when we arrived, and few of the patrons were as yet about. My companion shouted "Hello, Louis" as a form so huge appeared in the doorway I thought he would shove the door jambs out as he came through. My father was a big man, and my grandfather was bigger, but this man looked like them both in one. I was awed out of my senses. My friend introduced me and Louis smiled kindly when he was informed that I was one who practiced lifting weights. The big man just felt my hand and wrist and said, "Yes, you're a strong boy." I colored visibly at this kindness, and the rest of the night my fascinated gaze never left the herculean proportions of the colossal chest, and back and the arms upon which the sleeves were rolled. That was all I could see of him above the bar, and enough for one night. As the gathering grew the patrons became noisy and more boisterous with every drink. Everything talked about was strength and every word of it I devoured. Finally, "Come, Louis, let me see if I can move your arm tonight, I feel terribly strong," one burly fellow sang out happily. Louis strode up behind the bar facing the challenger with a smile and placed his huge arm upon the bar with the forearm bent at right angles. With both hands the burly fellow took hold of Louis' hand, and throwing all his weight backwards he tried to pull the iron arm down. It was useless. He reminded me of a fly dangling on the end of a fishing hook. Then he called for his friend to help him. Two more complied and all Louis did was to double up his forearm on the biceps to foil their resistance. At another time I saw Louis perform a feat by which he is commonly remembered. Men came from all over with the hope of witnessing this unusual stunt, and in it there was a great deal of secret tact between Louis and his wife. Though it was never said so, but I always believed it to be a trade-drawing stunt, and the way it was offered it was never meant to appear as a stunt, but more or less of a commonplace event in the order of their matrimonial life. Louis would be standing with arms folded on the bar, talking to the patrons (he was always talking when it happened), when from the rear Madame would emerge dressed for the street, and simply say "Louis." Without breaking his speech or taking his eyes away from their original object, one big arm would slide off the bar. Madame would then sit down upon the palm of that great platter of hand without doing anything other than pull on her gloves, or look into her handbag, while as easily and smoothly as the hoist of an elevator, her weight would be curled over the height of the bar, and then in a clear muscle- out, she would be transferred over the bar and gently lowered on the other side until her feet touched the floor. Sliding off the hand, she would then pass out into the street with the commonplace expression of one who had ordinarily used an elevator, or an escalator, to transfer them along from one place to another. Silence was the biggest attribute ever paid to this wonderful feat. Never was their any vociferous applause heard or resounding of clapped hands or stamped feet upon the floor. They spoke their thought to each other by shaking heads in an understanding way. While Louis continued his conversation, unmoved, a past master of showmanship.

The manner in which he loaded or unloaded barrels of beer and wine off the brewery trucks, would have excited the envy of Goliath. Three hundred and twenty pounds, four hundred; 'twas all alike to him. He grasped the barrel by the chines and with one swing hurled it onto the dray wagon or upon his one shoulder, as perfectly as if a windlass had been employed, and with it stride away with his long, heavy, measured tread, like a patrolling soldier on picket duty with shouldered rifle.

Here is a little stunt worth the telling which he used to do when he wore long hair which almost slipped my mind. In the folds of his twisted tresses he tied three fifty-pound weights, one on each side of the head and one in the center. With these dangling from his scalp, he would spin around until they whirled and whizzed like the propeller on an aeroplane. It always presented a thrilling sight and never failed to delight, and for years he used this stunt with which to wind up his act. But he later cut off his hair, and with it went this spectacular stunt.

As I have often said, Louis never refused a bet on odds of strength. Nor was he ever backward in working out a physical problem. Watching an engine drag a long line of freight cars through a station, he and his friends began to speculate on the weight of a freight car, and the relative amount of man power it would take to push one along. Louis exclaimed after a moment of thought, "I am willing to wager that I can push one along." Doubt was expressed by one of the group, and a wager was made. Cyr jumped right into the task by simply throwing off his coat. The hardest part was the start, but as those two under pins of power straightened themselves the car began to move. Steadily he pushed the car along, not on the level track but up a grade. Just the same, the pride of America had his limitations, and on two occasions he was worsted in the conflict. The first I will relate is amusing and also surprising. I bet if someone asked you if you could pass through the full length of a train and open and shut all the windows one after the other without a pause you would say you could. Louis said so, but he failed. His great strength played out just before he completed the round, and never has there been known a man to succeed in this task, no matter how used he is to the work, or how strong. This is one of those tests that on first hearing sounds as unbelievable as the ability to tie you up helpless with a foot of thread. Just as surely as the latter can be done, just as surely can the former not be done.

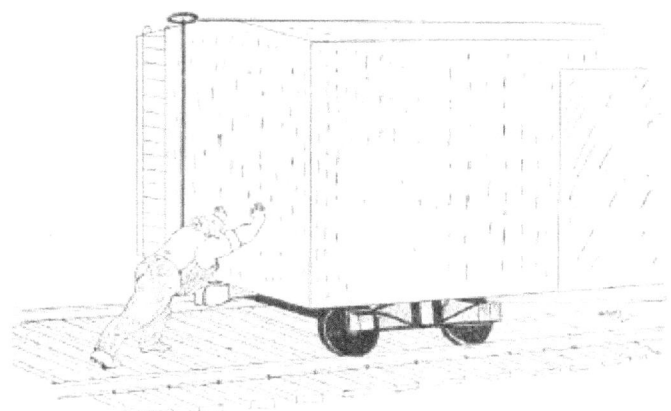

The second time that Louis got stumped was by a pure piece of trickery. I am willing to say if he had known it at the time things would have gone ill with the party concerned. It all happened in the Bowery of New York, where a big ex-strong man kept a saloon. This man boasted that no man was ever as strong as he, and on the floor of the saloon he had a huge weight placed between two low trestles that acted as a platform for each foot of the lifter to stand on. At the top of the weight was a large ring through which passed a heavy piece of straight iron that acted as a bar to lift the weight with. The object was to stand straddle of the weight by grasping the handle and lift. Something like a two-hand dead lift off the floor. This saloon proprietor had a standing wager that no man could lift it but he. From the very moment Louis heard of it he had a strong desire to see this stubborn piece of metal that would only raise to the exertion of one man. On the first opportunity he had, down to this Bowery saloon he went. The moment Louis walked in and saw the bloated appearance of a man smaller than he, he figured the lift was all over. The wager was accepted, and everybody gathered around to see the test. Louis stepped astride the mass of metal and began to lift, but not a move. He set himself and tried again, with no better result. Louis was astounded. He looked at the saloonkeeper and then at the weight, bewildered for the first time in his life. It made him angry, so that he grabbed the bar again and lifted till he saw stars, and the bar bent under the great pressure of his pull. Still the weight remained unmoved. Louis knew now that there was something phoney about it, but so skilfully was the trick concealed that he was not able to accuse the man of fraud. But in order to win the wager the saloonkeeper had to make the lift. Brazen from use, he arrogantly stepped from behind the bar, and with one pull lifted the weight clear off the floor.

Professor Adrian Schmidt was very familiar with the whole affair; he told me that he had often been around and seen the trick pulled off. But all things come to those who wait, and sure enough exposure came to this faker. The saloonkeeper had employed a darkey cellar helper and one day they came to words, and then to blows. The upshot was that the beaten-up smoke took some fellows in to see how the lifting trick was done. In the center of the weight was a tongue which passed through a hole in the floor. In the tongue was cut a slot through which a bar was put whenever a wager was made, a signal was sent down to the darkey, who kept the bar in when the other fellow tried. He always knew when the saloonkeeper was going to lift by the manner of his walk, which was also his cue to take out the bar. The other lifter would have to lift the floor up in order to move the weight, which you know is impossible. You might wonder why it was never detected, but it is not so easy to see clear underneath a wide, flat object that is only moved a half inch off the floor for a fraction of time and immediately dropped in order to make a lift.

Just another little story in which I was fooled, and where the superiority of our hero over the present-day great luminaries of the iron circle was proven.

You will remember me mentioning Professor Louis Attila in conjunction with Eugene Sandow. Well, Attila left Sandow when the latter decided to return to England after his American tour. The Professor started up himself on Broadway, New York, and his gymnasium became the meeting place of all great iron men as long as Attila ran it. It was in that place that Louis Cyr and Horace Barre always trained when they came to New York. When Louis retired he gave the Professor one of his bar bells as an appreciation for old times' sake. It weighed a little over one hundred and ninety pounds and has a thick handle which fits solidly into each sphere. This bell Louis snatched with one hand at every performance. It happened on one of my visits to Attila's gymnasium we were discussing Cyr and the remark was made that no man of all who had tried had ever snatched the bar once. I remarked that I thought if anyone could make the snatch lift with it, I believed that Henry Steinborn was the man. I was meeting Henry quite regularly then, and the next time I saw him I told him about it. Now I want you to bear in mind that Henry always figured that he was good enough for a one-hand snatch of two hundred and thirty pounds, and I had seen him do some wonderful stuff. A few days later we met again and he laughingly said, "Say, why did you tell them down at Attila's that I could lift that bell of Cyr's. They had me try it and I could do nothing with it." In surprise I said, "Honest." "Sure," he remarked, "the handle is so thick and the weight so dead I couldn't get it started, and I do not think anyone else can."

# CHAPTER VIII

Well, my friends and brother strength lovers, I am coming to the end of the career of this great wielder of the Titan rod. His saloon and farm interests began to call for more of his attention than ever, which finds him at the close of the nineteenth century completely retired from active show life. He still held the title along with the belt, but was thankful for the seclusion of domestic life, as is always true of a man who has wandered over the world for many years. Louis was a model husband, a good father and a great friend of every man. I am not saying this because I feel a great affection for him. It is one thing in me to admire a man for his talent, and another thing to admire him for his general principles. If he had any shortcomings other than commonly found in man I would say so, but I can honestly say that he was the only great athlete I never saw stones thrown at.

Curiously calm, he rarely showed anger even when under the sting of provocation. He was full of kindness and lived an exemplary life before the eyes of all who knew him. His courtesy never forsook him, for in him was all the chivalry of old France, and the hand of arrogance had never touched his brow. As a son of the soil he lived, with the kindred tastes that go with the people of the soil, which are so simple to fulfill. His fealty was now centered in his home, and on his wife and daughter. Although he had always loved his profession earnestly, and served the gods who rule the iron children faithfully and generously. In return they had smiled upon him and crowned his life with success and fortune. His home was a veritable palace of trophies, bestowed upon him at one time and another by his admirers, who ranged from the crowned heads of the world to the poorest plowman.

The first few years after 1900 passed away uneventfully, but Canada was still producing her remarkable quota of strong men, fast growing into manhood. About 1904 Louis began to show signs of failing health, due to his excessive eating and life of inactivity. His physical appearance had changed, and the body had become very corpulent, so that he would say it was easier for him to lift a ton than pick up a pin. Actually he weighed over four hundred pounds.

He seriously began to consider giving the title to some other worthy man of strength, but irrespective of his ill health, he said that whoever took it must take it in combat so that he would be proved worthy of the honor. In 1906 he agreed to meet Hector DeCarrie, a young Montrealer who had displayed remarkable ability, but way below what Cry could show at any time. Nevertheless, by popular opinion he was looked upon as the best bet on the American continent, since Barre had also retired. It so happened that around the time of the match Louis was in much poorer health than usual. In fact, he had not touched a weight for a long time, and actually done no steady training since his retirement. His physician begged of Louis not to engage in the contest, but the indomitable soul of Louis rose over the weakness of his flesh and he remained obdurate—lost in the heart of the little whispering voice of other days that was once again fanning the spark of conquest. They met at Sohmer Park, Montreal, but it was a sadly different Louis to the one who had defied the power of the horses fourteen years before in the eyes of a wildly cheering assemblage.

Louis sat down between every lift. Quite different to the vitallic, eager moving man who before was always impatient for his turn. The first lift was a one-hand press with feet together. Louis raised one hundred and fifty-one and one- half pounds and DeCarrie one hundred and seventy-one and one-half pounds, though the crowd hooted the lift of DeCarrie as improper, but Louis waved his assent to the judges to pass it. Cyr made a swing to arm's length overhead with the same weight, and DeCarrie refused to try it. Next they lifted a bell while sitting on a chair, using one hand. Cyr did one hundred and thirty-nine pounds against one hundred and fifty-one and one-half pounds by Hector. The crowd protested again, but Louis paid no attention to it, so they passed on to the next lift, which was a two-hand clean lift from the ground to the shoulder and then jerk overhead. The gallant veteran could hardly stand, but the unquenchable spirit of his fathers that had driven the murderous redskins before them rose within him, and he actually pressed two hundred and eighty-eight pounds. This the young challenger would not try.

I should have told you at the beginning that each man had picked four lifts, with the contest starting on Louis' choice. The finish of the set found Louis way ahead, with a total of seven hundred and thirty pounds against three hundred and twenty-three pounds. DeCarrie had only made two lifts out of the four. They next passed on to DeCarrie's set, commencing with a one-hand dumb bell-lift, which was won by DeCarrie by ten pounds; that is, two hundred and twenty pounds against two hundred and ten pounds. Then followed a two-dumb-bell lift. Louis pushed up two hundred and twenty-seven pounds, but DeCarrie could not make the grade and refused to try. Then they had a repetition lift with a one hundred and fifty-one and one-half pound dumb bell. Louis got in four presses against five by Hector. The final lift was a back lift which Louis easily won, doing two thousand eight hundred and seventy-nine pounds, a poundage which DeCarrie would not try.

Now in repetition lifting, which was quite a fad in those days with some, they would multiply the poundage by the number of times the object was lifted. Therefore on the dumb bell repetition lift, DeCarrie was credited with seven hundred and fifty-one and one-half pounds by lifting the weight five times. DeCarrie's set of four lifts was won by Louis with a total of three thousand nine hundred and twenty-two pounds against nine hundred and seventy-seven and one-half pounds. The grand total was four thousand six hundred and fifty- two pounds to Cyr with one thousand three hundred and one-half pounds to DeCarrie. This was his last act, and as the curtain was drawn over the scene it was to cover him as a winner, and a glorious victor. No wonder the sun set in glory as the last lift was made. The heavens flushed with victory and bathed the waning rays of the sun in gold and blood red—the gold of victory spilling its honors over the blood of a great warrior. Staggering and reeling, he closed the portals of his career in a triumph never equaled, and as he turned to leave he blessed the young man, on whom he transferred his title. Sickness could not rob him of victory, nothing living could, only death. But the precipice of life found him just the same bat- tling Louis as of old, calm and dignified.

He passed away at his home in Montreal on November 10th, 1912, with chronic nephritis. His death cast a great sadness oyer the royal city, and every bell tolled in reverence of her most distinguished son. All the Canadian newspapers carried huge black headlines announcing his demise, and the news shot around the world with the startling alacrity only equaled two years later, when the world throbbed at the news of the invasion of Belgium.

The ancient province went into mourning, and flags flew at half mast. He was buried in regal state by the Holy Catholic Church in a splendor of magnificence never shown to any gladiator in the history of the world. The pomp of state and church combined, and never was there a royal entourage more glorious than this, for the man who was just a strong man. Every street was packed with mourners all the way from the church to the "way of the cross."

A bare-headed multitude crowded the cemetery, and as the last funeral rites were performed at the graveside, the "Last Post" was sounded, and the muffled drums rolled out their thunder to mingle with the dying echo of the bugle, while the rifles barked out their last salute to the man who has been called "The Daddie of 'Em All," as a Godspeed to his great soul, as it ascended on the way to the halls of Valhalla, where the "Saga" stories tell us all the great gladiators are gathered.

The death of Sir Wilfred Laurier, Canada's most brilliant statesman and the man acclaimed by the world as the most brilliant orator of this generation, did not receive the same homage as paid to all that was left mortal of the great- souled Louis Cyr. It was the greatest and most magnificent spectacle ever seen in Montreal, where the magnitude of magnificence is outrivaled. This alone speaks louder than my pen can write of the life of the man, and the esteem in which he was held by all who knew him.

There are pessimists who point him out, and tell you all strong men die young. Bah! we should worry about what they say. All things happen for a purpose, and Cyr died because he was subject to the frailties of the flesh. He was only human, and he killed himself with gluttony, just as you and I would do if such was our weakness. I am making no excuses for him, neither have I cold feet that shake from facts, but I am human, so who am I to judge. Only fools and pessimists judge the death of a man. It is the life he led that counts, the good he did and the lesson he left. From the cradle to the grave the life of Louis Cyr was filled with usefulness. You know what the philosophy of the Arab says, "that man better live one score years and ten in usefulness than three score years and ten in indifference." Cyr did better than that. If nothing else, he left much in himself to be admired and little to be found fault with. What is it that Kipling says on the creed of man in that famous song of "The Seven Seas"?

"Only the Master shall praise us, and only the Master shall blame And no one shall work for money, and no one shall work for fame, But each for the joy of working, and each on his separate star Shall draw the things as he sees it for the God of Things as they are."


That is just what Cyr did, and what he did was done well and done honorably. It is true that behind the living we see the dead, but such a man is deathless, the kind that lives beyond the grave to spur us on to exemplify and extol the wonders of physical manhood by our own efforts and example.

A few months ago I called on Dr. Ammou, the husband of the charming daughter of the great sire, at their home in Montreal. Madame showed me her greatest treasure, the championship belt which her father had won and worn, and as he was never defeated it never passed away from him, but remains now a family heirloom. Madame Louis Cyr is still alive, and when mention is made of her great lord the color will mount to her cheeks and her eyes flash in honest pride. Louis may be gone, but she is still in love with him. Peter Cyr, the young brother of Louis, is alive and takes care of his farm that lies on the outskirts of Montreal, and he still takes a great deal of interest in the deeds of strong men, but loyal as they make 'em, he never will believe the world will produce another like the brother he worshipped. Horace Barre slipped out into the great beyond seven years after his great teammate, and so the story is told.

Last summer I made a pilgrimage to the shrine of the herculean monarch of Ironia, and as I stood by the side of his grave the leaves of time unfolded, and I read again the life of him who now is but a glorious memory. Like one body attracts another, I felt his great presence, and a wonderful happiness filled me, and I thanked God that such a man had lived. The next day I sailed away from Montreal on the swelling bosom of the majestic St. Lawrence. I watched the royal city through the dusk of the evening as the twilight veil of natural loveliness settled down, shrouding as it were, her great son, until the myriad stars broke out like little drops of jeweled silver, and I thought of what Spencer said of what constitutes our existence, Life, Space and Time. The Life to live, the Space to expand in, and the Time to do good in. Ah! Yes, most people could live a thousand years all for no purpose. But Louis Cyr exem plified those three gifts as no other man did, by his wonderful, forcible, indomitable strength, and an unquenchable spirit of fire that has blazed a trail in strongmanism never touched before or since. Never did such crowds gather to follow a man as they did him, and we still continue to follow him. Why Not? Millions worship the god of Gold and the flaming diamond. Then is it not nobler to worship the great gift of God—a glorified body with a glorified soul—which He fashioned and made, and placed as a beacon among men to impress us. To me, men like Cyr are the emancipators of clean living, that carry us nearer to the path of "the way to live" which so many blindly seek. But never has there been another who by his terrific strength and kindly smile, by his flaming spirit and honest heart proved himself to stand equal with the greatest of them all, Louis Cyr —the Great Canadian— "The Daddy of 'em all."

# REMINISCENCE

Some years ago I wrote an article entitled, "Quebec, The Cradle of Strong Men." The title was the result of a statement I had made in which I remarked that within the province of Quebec could be found the strongest men in the world. The statement, and the article, drew widespread interest and comment as to what was the cause of this apparently extraordinary condition among an approximate number of two million people. Was it diet, race or hereditary condition? That was the exact question raised in an editorial. I often turned that question over in my mind, but not for one moment did I consider the question of diet. I know only too well the thrifty frugal table of the habitant of Quebec, and while the table is well provided for the variety is scant. Three things which the dietitians taboo, namely, pork, white bread and maple syrup, they eat in abundance. The question of race might have something to do with it, but I very much doubt it.

The first people of Canada were the French Catholic Colonists, but very quickly they began to infuse the blood of the Huron and Iroquois into their progeny, and I doubt if there can be found a real native of Quebec wholly free of Indian blood. I say this in view of the fact that no person can call himself a true native unless he can produce a lineage of four generations on the native soil. The French Canadians can produce such an heritage more easily than the English Canadian. Through this race commingling we find the blood ties of New France separated from Old France, and along with the change of blood ties we find a diversity of language. In my estimation, there is all the difference in the world between the Frenchman of France, and the Frenchman of Canada, and it is also true that the native of Quebec recognizes this condition and does not recognize an absolute affinity with the old land. They grew as a race apart.

France refused to believe it, but when the famous French Canadian battalions first paraded through Paris enroute during the great war, it became an established reality to them. France was curious to look upon the descendants of the hardy followers of Cartier and Champlain, and well I remember the French papers commenting on their observations of the prodigals and saying that, "They found them different." If it had been a question of race they would not have been different. History is full of such incidents. The dispersion of the various Gothic nations as they trod underfoot the various civilizations in their barbarous conquests in the different parts of Europe proves this. They were in time absorbed by the conquered in a process of natural absorption. Most of these all-conquering Teuton races became Latinized. If these particular war-like races had within them the all-dominating features they would never have been absorbed. Other great nations fell of moral decay—for instance, the Hellenic Empire and the Empire of the Caesars. In only one instance have we any record of a race perpetuating its domination—the Anglo-Saxons. The Norman conquest of England was absorbed within one generation and the British race predominated as Anglo-Saxon.

Of hereditary conditions as a cause there probably are a few more reasons for belief, although I cannot bring myself to analyze this question in the same light as the masters of eugenics analyze hereditary traits, through their experiments with guinea pigs, white mice and rabbits. Whether I am right or wrong, I base my beliefs as history and ethnology have taught me, and until I am proved wrong I shall continue to believe that I am right.

It has always been a doubtful question in my mind as to just how much hereditary has to do with the success of a nation, but with an individual it is quite probably much more important. Yet the greatest fundamental that I have come to recognize is—environment. This condition more than any other makes men what they are. In itself it is the product of conditions or circumstances. The conditions and circumstances of Canada as found by its first settlers, were what determined the real hardiness of the future Canadian. Only the fittest survived, and necessity set for them a task of toil. It developed the true spirit of the pioneer, and from that such a man as Louis Cyr sprung. Among them, strength is a natural acquisition, they do not look for it, they expect it, and taking great pride in the amount they exhibit, the element of combat evolved.

Louis Cyr is not the only great man Quebec had, there are many others, but the great Louis was the greatest of them all. Further investigations proved that Louis was advertising the fact that in the same province were other men of powerful bone and sinew, more capable of comparison with himself than some of the luminaries of Europe. Louis had already produced the prodigious Horace Barre, a man who had on several occasions shouldered a bar bell of twelve hundred and seventy pounds, and carried it the entire length of the gymnasium on each occasion.

Imagine a bar bell of twelve hundred and seventy pounds—would you not believe that such a weight on a bar would not only overbalance a man so that it would be impossible for him to carry it, but the weight on the bar would cause it to be buried deep into the flesh of the shoulder so that the burden would be unbearable. But Barre did it. Twice he performed the feat in the gymnasium of Professor Attila, in New York, and on other occasions in Montreal. Doing the feat so often is evidence enough that it was not his record performance. He could have done more.

Just the direct opposite was little Bourette, a man who did not weigh much over one hundred pounds stripped. The little dynamo teamed with Louis in his circus troupe, and at every performance he raised a huge bar bell to arms length that weighed two hundred and thirty pounds, while lying on his back. I met Bourette years after his retirement when he was in his fifties, and he could still do it, although he had not touched a weight for years. He performed part of a tremendous spectacular feat with Louis, in which the iron king held a bar bell in his hands, on which Bourette would hang suspended with his hocks. Then Louis, quite matter of fact, would raise the combined weight to his shoulders, and push the weight out straight in front so that his arms were straight, and level with the shoulder. Slowly, he would return the man and weight to the shoulders. It seems terribly hard for the layman to believe a front "muscle out" like that, but it was just a routine feat for the king of strength.

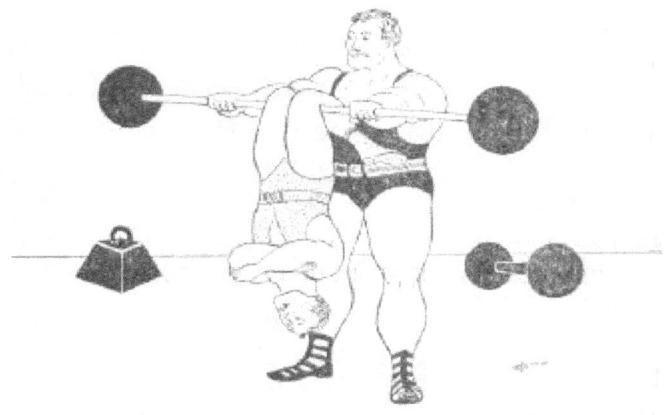

Then again, remember his brother, Peter, as a lad of nineteen was invincible as a middle weight. All at one time we find four supermen produced from a population that then numbered not much over a million people. It was environment that created them, but it was Louis that created the environment. He inspired others, and they accustomed themselves to consider certain poundages as being ordinary, that really shocked the best products of other nations. Well, we always follow a leader and usually find that the magnitude of his brilliance is a cause for our continued striving. The brilliancy of Leader Louis was that he daily reduced the extraordinary in feats of man power to the commonplace.

These points that I have just covered were accepted by all those who had become deeply interested in this topic, but you know how one question will raise another. They pondered over the thought whether Quebec would always be the cradle of strong men. That is something that will always rest upon the lap of the gods. It all depends upon how time will affect the people of Quebec, and whether the future generation will be caught in the whirligig of fast life or not. So far these people have remained much to themselves, clannish if you wish to use the term, but free of the bigoty that prevails over most clannish races. They choose their bosom friends, and their wives from amongst themselves because they feel a closer relationship. It is not hate that separates them from others, but a greater affection for their own. We have to admire them for that.

Anyhow the march of progress has lifted all new countries far away from the pioneer days, which is also true of Quebec, and still we find the Anglo-French colony true to her Titan traditions. Of the men who followed Louis, perhaps the most notable was the young Montrealer, Hector DeCarrie. He certainly was a real good man, but lacked much of the bodyweight that Cyr and Barre had. I doubt if he ever made the two hundred pound bodyweight mark. Of course, we do not hear anything of DeCarrie now, as he retired from the strong man profession some years ago. Like all French Canadian strong men he was great on separate dumb-bell lifting, and he was a wonder on the bent press. He actually claimed to be the first man to do over three hundred pounds with one hand. Be that as it may, DeCarrie was the best man in Canada for many years. Then came Wilfred Cabana, who before he was out of his teens forged to the front with some stupendous claims, but he never conclusively proved his superiority over DeCarrie. Cabana became the rage. He was a regular Adonis, and it looked as though he was going to revive the old glories that had passed away with the incomparable Louis, but lack of proper management, and the refusal to be true to himself lost him his popularity, and he never climbed far on the steps that led to fame. Cabana was really ingenious, and contrived some wonderful feats, but his actual lifting was based upon his bent press ability. I remember quite well his human bridge stunt, performed a la Strongfort. Unfortunately he was badly injured when the driver of the automobile lost control of the machine, which brought the whole works down upon him. LaVallee was the next superman that invaded the field. He was undoubtedly the most powerful man since the days of Cyr. Of him I have written considerably in "The Key to Might and Muscle." Here was a man I would dearly have liked to seen featured. He was of a tremendous stature, tall, and well put together with enormous girth of limb. He reminded me much of Apollon, the old French idol, whom he resembled in every way, even to the extent of his laziness in being unwilling to demonstrate the actual limit of his strength.

Around this time there sprung up another who claimed much public attention, Victor DeLamarre. He came from further east in the province, but to be frank with all my brother strength lovers, I cannot say that this man was in the same class as any of the other men I have mentioned on pure strength tests. He is a fine showman, but that is all, and I merely mention him because so many interested parties have written to me concerning him. From the moment I first saw him perform at the St. Dennis Theatre, in Montreal, I did not take him seriously. I do not think that he weighs over one hundred and sixty pounds, and I feel quite sure that Fourneir could easily dispose of him on any set of lifts.

At that time, I could have put my hands on a dozen men in Montreal alone, who collectively, could defeat the twelve best men all the other nations of the world put together could bring. Since then, the world has made rapid strides in the strength field, and developed some wonderful material. Nevertheless, Quebec still produces the quota from her handful, that can challenge the world on an even footing.

I quite expect that there are some who will be inclined to think that Quebec's production is an accident. They may think that a province of so small a population could not lord it over the rest of the world otherwise. Now here is where I want you to understand me thoroughly. I am not one who puts things down to miracles or accidents, when anything unusual becomes repeated more than two or three times. There is always a reason to be found somewhere, is my belief. It is not because the French Canadians are a northern people that they are so sturdy. The Scandinavian races have a similar climate, but they, as a people do not compare with the Canadian strong men. It is all in environment, the atmosphere we live in that moulds our character and disposition. Quebec is not the only country that has proved this. Look at little Esthonia and the powerful men it lias produced. They claim George Hacken- schmidt, Lurich and Aberg of the old regime, and are responsible for such splendid men as Neuland, Kikkas and Tammer of the present day. It is an Estonian strength club that has the highest standard of any other club in the world. No man over one hundred and eighty- two pounds is admitted into membership, who cannot make a two hands jerk in two clean movements of three hundred pounds. I am aware of the fact that Hackenschmidt, Lurich and Aberg have claimed Russia as their nationality, but then, Esthonia was part of Russia. On the other hand it was easier for them to say they came from Russia, just the same as it is for a native of Quebec to say he is from Canada.

It has been environment with Esthonia, as with Quebec, that has developed such a high standard, and kept it, and as long as they cater to strength as their national sport, each nation will continue to produce extraordinary specimens.

Montreal has been the scene of many rare strength fests, and seen many a great man come and go. Last summer Arthur Giroux retired, and with him went much of that which we admire in the man of bone and sinew. He was a popular national figure, and endeared himself to the hearts of many American strength lovers. He did not commence to display his powers until he was thirty-four years of age, and when he did, he made them all step. I never knew a lifter who was as anxious as he was to satisfy others as to the honesty of the weights that he lifted. In that respect he was like his great forerunner, Louis Cyr. He was exceptionally good at walking with weights in both hands, and naturally his grip was unusually strong. He held the beautiful national trophy from the French Canadian Federation of Weight Lifters, for many years, turning it in during the summer of 1926, when he announced his retirement.

Arthur Dandurand was also a fine speciman of manhood, and among the smaller men, Fournier, Marineau, Angers, Gratton, and Bar- beau are wonders. But Montreal has recently brought to light another figure whose calibre of strength surpasses that of any other since the advent of Cyr. His name is Caouette. He is not yet thirty years of age, but is an enormous man, heavier even than Cyr. He strips at three hundred and fourty-seven pounds, but is so powerful that it is hard to give any exact estimate of his strength at the present time. On some feats he equals the great Louis, but whether he can equal him on all the tests, or beat him, is something that remains to be proved.

I have known them all, along with many others whom I have not mentioned, and with due respect to them all, including the powerful new comer, Caouette, none of them come within a thousand miles of touching the great Louis. With the exception of De Lavalee and Caouette, not one of them had anywhere near the strength of Cyr. Even if they had, there was many things that Cyr had, which they lack. This can be equally applied to all the strong men of any other country. Cyr was magnetic. He attracted, and swayed the public with his inborn traits of showmanship that was brought to the peak of perfection, from use. A promoter who had handled Louis, told me that he was the easiest man in the world to handle. He was a shrewd business man, but never exorbitant, and at no time was he known to resort to harsh words. Louis would say what he had to say, and if they could not agree on terms, well, there was no harm done. They all could part with a handshake, knowing Louis was still a friend. Most men who rise to the peak that Louis reached, are as hard to handle as any operatic star—No wonder their managers die young.—

I have never met a strong man from the land of the maple leaf who did not feel that Louis was something way beyond the rest of them.

Dear old Montreal, it has always been the Mecca of strong men on this side of the Atlantic, and rivals such great centers as Munich, Vienna and Reval. American traditions have reposed in the old city of Boston, although during the last few years, Philadelphia has become the hub of attraction. Even so, Boston still retains some magnificent characters. In Louis' days, it was the place and became more popular because the great king of fistiania commenced his career and lived his life there. John L. Sullivan was the first known to the sporting public as—"The Boston Strong Boy," and throughout his life he was tremendously proud of his strength. It was the feature of his ring career. Never was he known to refuse a test with any man of brawn, and he claimed no man was as strong as he unless he proved it. Incidentally, John L. had some pet stunts all of his own that really took some doing, but he found all his best as nothing against the superior powers of Our Louis.

These two men were very friendly, although John L. was very repugnant to Louis when John was under the influence of drink, which was very often. While much can be said for John L. as a fighter, and much for him as a man, when sober, nevertheless when drinking he was degraded. He reigned with a rule of terror, and it is a fact that when he called for every man to drink to his toast, he drank. He pulled this stunt off wherever he went, and always when the bar room was the most crowded. His voice was the roar of a bull, and as loud as he could roar he would call for everyone to line up against the bar. This done, and with everyone standing glass in hand waiting for the toast, John L. would exclaim, 'Here's to John L. Sullivan, I can lick any son of a ----- in the world." As they drank, Sullivan would glare around from under his scowling brow to see if anyone had not responded. The day came when one man did refuse, none other than Louis Cyr. They had both walked into a saloon, and when the crowd had gathered to its largest, John L. made his usual boastful toast. The glass was to the mouth of Louis when the speech began, but as it progressed a look of reproach settled upon his face, and he returned his glass to the bar. Sullivan had drank enough to bring all the viciousness of his nature to the surface, which always laid dormant when he was sober. "Drink!" he roared out at Louis, but Louis just shook his head. "I'm sorry, M'sier, I cannot drink to that. Not that I question you as the best fighter in the world, but you should not use that expression." Silence settled upon all as tense as that experienced by a soldier waiting for a flying bomb to explode. John was shocked speechless for the moment, but he quickly recovered and took a step closer to Louis, with the glass in his hand that Louis had set down.

"Drink that!" he shouted, almost purple in the face, but Louis replied by placing one hand on John L.'s chest, and gave him a push that sent the drunken prize fighter reeling up against the bar. That was all. Sullivan then came to his senses, and manfully said to Louis, "I did not mean it that way, Louis." The breach thus filled, Louis called for drinks all round, and toasted—"To the champion fighter of the world, John L. Sullivan," to which everyone there applauded, glad to be released from the tense situation. This little incident alone proves Louis' broadness of mind. Some men with half the strength that Cyr had would have tried to have taken advantage of the situation. Instead, Louis gave John L. a chance to reassert himself, which he did. Judged in our day, such a statement is a deep affront, and most men are likely to resent it. Many years ago it was used as an expression of deep friendship, or in terms of admiration, but with it went the cowboy's advice, "Say, pard, when yuh use that name, smile." John L. Sullivan never smiled, his face always bore a ferocious scowl with which he always tried to reduce his opponent.

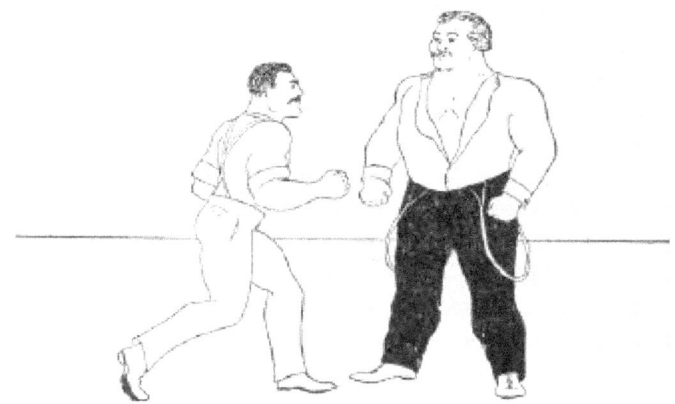

However, that expression broke a friendship later on that ended in a thrashing being administered to him by James J. Corbett, who also took his title. Cyr and Corbett are the only two men known who had dared to refuse the toast to Sullivan and get away with it. Cyr did not pass the thing off lightly because he was afraid of Sullivan. Not a bit. Cyr quite well knew that John L. was supposed to be most dangerous when under the influence of drink. Louis was positively fearless, and as I have stated in the first chapter of this book, Cyr could outfight any man in the province. Of course, that meant in a rough and tumble fight, hitting when down, as well as when up. John L. came to think an awful lot of Cyr, and he would laugh heartily at his vain attempts to move the arm of Louis in a wrist- turning test. On one of these impromptu occasions John L. said, "I bet I can hit a harder blow than you, Louis. Big as you are, I can knock you off your feet with a blow on the chest." To this Louis replied, "No, John, you can't." "By Hokey, I can," John declared, and each man rose to his feet. "All ready," John L. asked. "Stand well back, boys, so you can catch him as he falls, or open the door wide, for I'm going to knock him for a row." Louis stood up squarely upon his feet, one foot braced ahead of the other, and his enormous chest thrust out a big enough target for a blind man to hit. John L. had rolled up the sleeve of his shirt after discarding his coat, and he measured his distance with the practiced eye of a fighter who is used to measure off an opponent for a blow. The Boston bruiser looked formidable enough as he drew back his powerful right arm to the shoulder and launched forward the blow with all the strength of his body behind. His fist struck with the thudding boom of a big dud shell as it buries its force in the earth. The onlookers gasped and exclaimed, as the contact of knuckles on breast bone collided, and resounded throughout the room. But the mountain of bone and muscle was not moved from off his feet. Sullivan was the most amazed man there; he had never dreamt that any man could physically repulse a blow of his. Ruefully he rubbed his hand and said, "Darn it all, Louis, I would not want to be pounding men like you in the ring."

There was one stunt in particular that was a favorite with John L. which he was everlastingly having fun with. He had a glass a little taller than the ordinary drinking glass, and also with a smaller circumference. In it he placed a silver dollar and challenged the onlookers to try and blow it out. It takes some doing, and very few have I seen do it. The object is to blow the breath as forcibly as possible into the glass, and see if the reaction of the air striking the bottom of the glass will lift the silver dollar out of the glass. John L. could do it every time, and as is to be expected, he stuck Louis for the stunt. It strikes me as funny that John L. should entertain the thought that Louis could not do as good as he. Goodness sake! A man with a sixty-inch chest surely has a pair of lungs in proportion, and the way Louis blew that silver dollar out was enough to make believe he had four pair of lungs within him. How that made John L. laugh. At another time they both were feeling exceptionally playful, and they decided to have a free-for-all bout. They donned the mitts, and John socked the big man of might as he charged in, but it could not stop him, and the next thing John knew was that he was being squeezed to death with two great arms that wrapped around his head like the tentacles of an octopus. John could not strike, and the next thing he was thrown to the ground with Louis on top. John L. thought the house had fallen on him, and big as Sullivan was, he was completely submerged in the gigantic folds of the giant that held him crushed and powerless. You can hardly believe that men of such size would feel inclined to indulge in such horseplay, but there was much of the boy in both of them. Boston never forget Louis any more than it ever forgot John L., and their popularity is what made their separate centers so famous in sport.

This retrospect has given me the opportunity to tell you a little more of Our Hero and of others who played a part with him, as well as of those inspired by the great iron master who followed after him. I have explained only in a brief way why I believe environment is the real cause of the success of Quebec. I did not see any reason to go into the technicalities of eugenics, or of history, for I do not think you are so deeply concerned with those subjects as much as you are in the evidence produced by the strength of the men we honor.

Lifting weights to the French Canadian is like cricket to the English and baseball to the American. It is their sport. Of course, strength covers a much wider field than the national sports I have mentioned do. Strength embraces the world and has lovers everywhere. Beyond a doubt it is because of the great scope it covers that so many questions and comparisons are raised. Some people like to talk about the wonderful physique of the South American Indians, who live in the high altitude of the Andes, or of the Zulu, the west Australian native of the interior, and so on. To me they mean nothing. The South American sickens.and dies when he descends from his high altitude, and the Australian when he comes in contact with the white. They can only live under certain conditions. Then they are not wholly physically strong. Give me the man that can go anywhere, and meet anyone on equal terms, and still remain strong. He holds our answer. Not these people who seclude themselves in the isolated spots of the earth.

We worship Louis Cyr because he was so much all man. It is for these characteristics that make up that type of men we prefer to follow him, and hold him, as our inspiration. If I had the wealth of some men, I would set up a monument to his glory, and in letters of gold inscribe the lesson he gave to manliness and clean living so that all who read would pause and check up on themselves. Show them the value of taking a personal physical inventory so that they would gladly throw away their vices and follow him, as you and I are doing, for the betterment of ourselves and our children.